Critical Issues in
Mental Health

Edited by

Robert Tummey and Tim Turner

palgrave
macmillan

First published 2008 by
PALGRAVE MACMILLAN

Palgrave Macmillan in the UK is an imprint of Macmillan Publishers Limited,
registered in England, company number 785998, of Houndmills, Basingstoke,
Hampshire RG21 6XS.

Palgrave Macmillan in the US is a division of St Martin's Press LLC,
175 Fifth Avenue, New York, NY 10010.

Palgrave Macmillan is the global academic imprint of the above companies
and has companies and representatives throughout the world.

Palgrave® and Macmillan® are registered trademarks in the United States,
the United Kingdom, Europe and other countries.

ISBN-13: 978–0–230–00905–9
ISBN-10: 0–230–00905–0

This book is printed on paper suitable for recycling and made from fully
managed and sustained forest sources. Logging, pulping and manufacturing
processes are expected to conform to the environmental regulations of the
country of origin.

A catalogue record for this book is available from the British Library.

Printed in Great Britain by the MPG Books Group, Bodmin and King's Lynn

Dedicated to my mother, Dilys:
Cara 'm Cymraeg Fam. Anrhegaist 'm buchedd
RT

For my mother Ann,
and in memory of my father, Mike Turner
TT

Contents

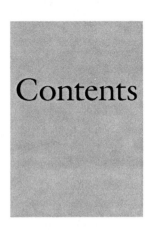

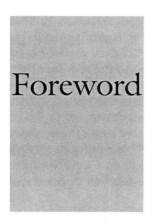

Foreword

It is a pleasure to provide a brief foreword to this edited volume by Bob Tummey and Tim Turner.

During the twentieth century, the idea that psychiatric disorders are diseases of the nervous system drove the delivery of mental health services throughout the industrialized West, and increasingly in the developing world also. A cursory inspection of any major psychiatric journal would give the impression that this development has been supported by advances in genetics and the neurosciences. Its consequence has been an increasing reliance on medical remedies for unhappiness and deviant behaviour. For example, in recent years there has been an escalating use of antidepressant drugs throughout the developed world (National Center for Health Statistics, 2006), and a similar rise in the use of antipsychotics, which are now not only administered to people with psychosis but to misbehaving children and the intellectually disabled (Olfson *et al.*, 2006) and sometimes to individuals thought to be at risk of severe mental illness (McGlashan *et al.*, 2006).

Despite these trends, the apparent triumph of biological psychiatry has owed more to political and financial interests than to science (Angell, 2004; Moncrieff, 2003). The evidence that psychiatric disorders are caused exclusively by biological rather than social factors is very poor (Bentall, 2003). Antidepressants, although ruthlessly marketed by the pharmaceutical industry (Lacasse and Leo, 2005), turn out to be hardly more effective than placebos (Kirsch *et al.*, 2008). Antipsychotics have side effects that can be severely threatening to physical health and, although alleviating distress in the short term, may have no long-term benefits (Bola, 2006). In contrast to other areas of medicine, in which progress has led to quantifiable improvements in prognosis (it was better to have a heart attack in 2001 than it was in

1901), modern psychiatric patients are more likely to be disabled (Whitaker, 2005) and are more likely to commit suicide than their Victorian counterparts (Healy *et al.*, 2006). Whereas medical services in the developed world ensure better outcomes than in the non-industrialized nations (it is better to have your heart attack in London than rural India), the opposite is the case for psychiatric conditions (Jablensky *et al.*, 1992).

Despite these dismal observations, many people working in mental health seem blind to the limitations of medical psychiatry. The anti-psychiatry movement of the 1960s and 1970s is a vague memory in the minds of most mental health professionals (when giving a lecture to a group of trainee clinical psychologists recently, I was shocked to discover that not a single student could tell me who R.D. Laing was).

This book therefore provides a welcome balance to the uncritical view of psychiatry that pervades our society today. Tummey and Turner have gathered together a distinguished group of authors, who have provided critical but clear and well-reasoned chapters covering a wide range of issues of importance to us all. It is a book that will be useful to both undergraduates contemplating careers in mental health, and trainees in the mental health professions. Hopefully, it will also attract the attention of the increasing number of ordinary people who are concerned about the state of our mental health services.

RICHARD BENTALL
Professor of Clinical Psychology and Neuropsychology,
University of Bangor

References

Angell, M. (2004) *The Truth About Drug Companies: How They Deceive Us and What to Do About It*. New York: Random House.

Bentall, R.P. (2003) *Madness Explained: Psychosis and Human Nature*. London: Penguin.

Bola, J.R. (2006) Medication-free research in early episode schizophrenia: evidence of long-term harm? *Schizophrenia Bulletin* 32: 288–96.

Healy, D., Harris, M., Tranter, R., Gutting, P., Austin, R., Jones-Edwards, G., *et al.* (2006) Lifetime suicide rates in treated schizophrenia: 1875–1924 and 1994–1998 cohorts compared. *British Journal of Psychiatry* 188: 223–8.

Jablensky, A., Sartorius, N., Ernberg, G., Anker, M., Korten, A., Cooper, J.E., *et al.* (1992). Schizophrenia: manifestations, incidence and course in different cultures. *Psychological Medicine* Supp 20: 1–97.

Kirsch, I., Deacon, B.J., Huedo-Medina, T.B., Scoboria, A., Moore, T.J. and Johnson, B.T. (2008). Initial severity and antidepressant benefits: a meta-analysis of data submitted to the food and drug administration. *PLoS Medicine* 5.

Lacasse, J.R. and Leo, J. (2005). Serotonin and depression: a disconnect between the advertisements and the scientific literature. *PLoS Medicine* 2: e392.

McGlashan, T.H., Zipursky, R.B., Perkins, D., Addington, J., Miller, T., Woods, S.W., *et al.* (2006). Randomized, double-blind trial of olanzapine versus placebo in patients prodromally symptomatic for psychosis. *Archives of General Psychiatry* 163: 790–9.

Moncrieff, J. (2003). *Is Psychiatry for Sale?* London: Institute of Psychiatry.

National Center for Health Statistics (2006) *Health, United States, 2006, with Chartbook of Trends in the Health of Americans*. Hyattsville, MD: US Government Printing Office.

Olfson, M., Blanco, C., Liu, L., Moreno, C. and Laje, G. (2006). National trends in the outpatient treatment of children and adolescents with antipsychotic drugs. *Archives of General Psychiatry* **63**: 679–85.

Whitaker, R. (2005). Anatomy of an epidemic: psychiatric drugs and the astonishing rise of mental illness in America. *Ethical Human Psychology and Psychiatry* 7: 23–35.

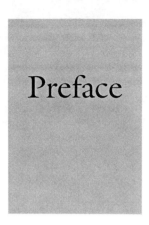

Preface

This book has been a while in the making, with one obstacle or another to overcome. We persevered through a number of personal triumphs and challenges to reach this point. The book prevailed and is now here for the reader to enjoy and absorb.

Our message is simple, but nonetheless important. Although tremendous strides have been made in mental health care, there is no room for complacency. In the abstract world of psychiatry it is essential that practitioners work reflexively. We need to recognise the negative forces that can influence our position. Each contributor to the book has written from a critical perspective based upon a wealth of clinical and academic knowledge. We hope you enjoy the contentious nature of a text that we believe makes an important contribution to the literature. Enjoy.

R.T.
T.T.

Acknowledgements

We are extremely grateful to a number of people who helped make this book a reality and supported the process from the beginning, especially Lynda Thompson and the team at Palgrave Macmillan. A special mention of thanks goes to the reviewers for their informative comments. Also, the people who offered help, interest and encouragement, including Tony Colombo, Douglas MacCarrick and Helen Poole at Coventry University and Judy Kilpatrick and Carole Schneebeli at the University of Auckland. Thanks to our friends and colleagues who provided support during our own critical issues: Steve Coniff, Ashley Crump, Andrew Davies, Michael Fenton, Mark Locke and Guy Powell; Jane Barrington, Jack Killingray and Rose Killingray, Patte Randall, Val Williams, Maurice Wogan and Elaine Wogan.

Most of all, love to Francesca, Hannah and Rhys; and Katherine, Sebastian, Scarlett and Jude, who make it all worthwhile.

Notes on Contributors

Professor Phil Barker is Honorary Professor at the University of Dundee, Scotland.

Poppy Buchanan-Barker is Director of Clan Unity International, Fife, Scotland.

Dr Anthony Colombo is Senior Lecturer in Criminology in the Department of Social and Community Studies at Coventry University, England.

Vicki Coppock is Reader in Social Work and Mental Health at Edge Hill University, Ormskirk, Lancashire, England.

Dr David T. Evans is Senior Lecturer in the Department of Sociology, Anthropology and Applied Social Sciences at the University of Glasgow, Scotland.

Dr Derek P. Farrell is Lecturer in Mental Health at the College of Medicine, Dentistry and Health Sciences, University of Birmingham, England.

Professor Suman Fernando is Honorary Senior Lecturer in Mental Health, European Centre for Study of Migration and Social Care (MASC) at the University of Kent, Canterbury, England and Visiting Professor in the Department of Applied Social Sciences at London Metropolitan University, London, England. Web site http://www.sumanfernando.com

Dr Lesley Henderson is Deputy Director of the Centre for Media, Globalisation and Risk and Lecturer in Sociology and Communications in the School of Social Sciences at Brunel University, Uxbridge, West London, England. Web site http://www.brunel.ac.uk/about/acad/sssl/ssslstaff/commStaff/LesleyHenderson

Professor Lucy Johnstone is Clinical Psychologist, Counselling Psychologist and currently Academic Director of the Bristol Clinical Psychology Doctorate at Bristol University, England.

David Pilgrim is Professor of Mental Health Policy at the University of Central Lancashire, Preston, England.

Anne Rogers is Professor of the Sociology of Health Care Primary Care Group, School of Community Medicine, in the Faculty of Medicine at the University of Manchester, England.

Francesca Tummey is Regional Development Worker for Child and Adolescent Mental Health Services at Care Services Improvement Partnership West Midlands, Birmingham, England.

Robert Tummey is Course Director and Senior Lecturer in Mental Health Nursing in the Department of Social and Community Studies, Coventry University, England.

Tim Turner is Senior Lecturer in Criminology in the Department of Social and Community Studies at Coventry University, England and a Registered Intermediary for the Ministry of Justice.

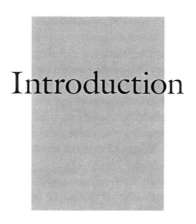

Introduction

Robert Tummey and Tim Turner

This book has come together gradually over a couple of years. The original idea arose as a result of an informal discussion decrying the absence of a good critical mental health text to inform a pre-registration nursing module called *Current Challenges in Mental Health*. Hopefully, this text addresses that absence by exploring key issues that are often either taken for granted or simply overlooked. The critical nature of the book is undoubtedly enhanced by the quality, reputation and imagination of the chapter authors, who represent some of the fiercest critics in the field.

The diverse, multifaceted nature of mental health care is reflected throughout the chapters, with a range of disciplinary perspectives and experiences represented. There is no dominant agenda or professional discourse. The pages that follow are written with a common theme: to question, critique and develop current mental health practice. This book is not intended as an inflammatory exposé; nevertheless important questions are raised that warrant discussion and reflection. The authors concerned have cast a critical eye over practice that is often blind, complacent and abusive. The central message of the text is a simple one: practitioners must critically reflect on their own practice in the wider context of a system that affords them considerable power in their work with vulnerable people.

While there is a wealth of critique here, this is not a negative text. Each of the chapters strives to move practice forward in a way that empowers service users and promotes recovery.

The book opens with a chapter that addresses an issue at the epicentre of mental health critique: psychiatric diagnosis. A critical appraisal of the medical model ensues with particular emphasis on the damaging impact on both service users and clinicians alike. While diagnosis provides a medical framework that can bring relief and understanding, it can also be construed as a negative label that consumes identity and dehumanizes the individual. Alternatives are explored through the concept of formulation, a psychological identification of influence that attempts to consider the individual in their own world and how they perceive that world. A balanced critical debate is provided that sets the tone for the proceeding chapters.

Chapters 3 and 8 specifically explore the impact of the service on the user. Chapter 3 takes a look at institutional racism in mental health care, by determining how race and culture impact on treatment provision. Attitudes and misrepresentations can be ingrained from generation to generation. Ignorance of culture and racial context paves the way for a recipe of uncertainty and fear in the shape of xenophobia. This phobia is a real fear experienced by society and mental health practitioners who live in that society. People of a different race, culture and religion endure prejudice and persistent discrimination. Sometimes the process is extremely vivid and overt; at other times it is subtle and covert. The innate undercurrent of racism that can occur in the institution is uncovered. It may cause concern to accept that such experiences still occur, but this chapter reveals the reality of what can and what does take place.

Like institutional racism, iatrogenic abuse is also embedded within service provision, through attitude, delivery and service-user experience. Chapter 8 is an attempt to provide the reader with an understanding of the daily risk of abuse that service users can experience. Many people who provide mental health care do not intend to abuse. However, circumstances can develop to 'overpower' the person, minimize their options, create barriers to their progress and use the platform of the medical model to medicate and incarcerate. On a micro-level, such practice may not be construed as abusive, but the use of force, gangs of staff, restraint, seclusion, medicating and so on can all too often spill into something non-therapeutic. Mental health care provision should be open to scrutiny and justification.

Such scrutiny is of course now commonplace within the media, which forms the focus of chapter 12. The mass media's role in exacerbating stigma through stereotypical images of mental illness is thoroughly explored. Various forms of media are placed under critical scrutiny to determine where poor portrayals have occurred. Positive media influences on public perception are also considered.

Through the context of exploring expression, chapter 4 on spirituality and chapter 5 on sexuality detail an interesting exploration of two areas that are frequently overlooked. Both stir up strong personal opinion in people and tend to be the subject of avoidance or ridicule. Spirituality is beautifully examined through a well-crafted amble of discovery and understanding, asking the question of its reality and context for individuals and clinicians by developing a philosophical stance, whereas sexuality highlights the variations of sexual orientation, the constraints on expression, the damage by institutions and general lack of mature, responsible debate within mental health care. The chapter unfolds to challenge the status quo and consider possible ways to move forward.

Two chapters that explore the reality of life experiences for people with mental illness are chapter 6 on gender and chapter 7 on the lifespan. The first identifies the disparity between care and treatment across gender. This subject considers whether being male or female delivers a different course of action and involvement and, ultimately, how this impacts on the perception of those responsible for treatment. This leads into chapter 7, which explores the evidence and perception of how mental illness affects people throughout the lifespan. It takes a look at how age influences the treatment offered and a person's susceptibility to differing forms of illness and diagnoses across the mental health spectrum. This interesting chapter maps the journey undertaken from the cradle to the grave. It is a fascinating elaboration of the stages and phases that mark a passage of time compatible with varying mental health issues.

Chapter 2 continues the exploration of life experiences by detailing the influence of socioeconomic disadvantage for mental health populations. The text provides an insight into the very real experience of those who exist on the margins of society who have limited empowerment and who can experience a genuine sense of injustice. The chapter unfolds as a critically informed narrative and is written from a position of academic authority.

The three chapters that remain focus attention on issues that preoccupy many contemporary practitioners and which are likely to dominate the future mental health landscape. The issue of risk is addressed in chapter 10, with a sociological context used to contextualize the current risk preoccupation within mental health care. The chapter invites practitioners to reflect on their role as risk assessors. This leads to the penultimate chapter 11, with an analysis of the complex relationship between mental health and crime. The chapter draws upon rich case examples of law to bring crime and mental illness to life. The distinct positions of both crime and risk in mental health care do not necessarily go hand in hand but both reflect the preoccupation with the unpredictable nature of mental illness.

The final chapter yet to be discussed is chapter 9, which provides an examination of psychological trauma. This takes a critical look at the historical context of trauma, its origins, its development and its presentation within a cynical world of litigation and blame. These may be unavoidable in the aftermath of a trauma, but can prolong distress and dictate the progress of the individual. Of course, litigation can be a relief for many, but not even an option for others.

Because of the nature of this book, each chapter is critical and contentious. Some of the issues covered are taboo and many of the questions raised may provoke practitioners to critically reflect on their role in terms of what they do, whom they do it for and what the implications are for those on the receiving end of treatment. We are aware that using terms such as abuse and racism in the context of care is controversial but we stand by their use, and at the very least hope that their inclusion stimulates debate. Throughout the book, the terms 'patient', 'client' and 'service user' are used interchangeably. This is due to the diversity of contribution, specific reference and the fact that no one term, as yet, is a 'catch-all' title that applies to all situations. Where possible, the term 'person' has been used.

1

Psychiatric Diagnosis

Lucy Johnstone

BRIEF CHAPTER OUTLINE

This chapter explores the purposes of psychiatric diagnosis and argues that theoretical justification is entirely lacking. A brief history is given consideration, leading through to contextualizing what diagnosis actually is. There are consequences of psychiatric diagnosis for both psychiatry and the service user. These are identified within a critique of the impact that psychiatric diagnosis has. International perspectives are given a succinct overview, which leads to a future vision. Here a response is offered for an alternative formulation approach as well as other categorization and naming.

Introduction

Why is the issue of diagnosis so important, both to the theory and practice of psychiatry and to any critical account of psychiatry? Although it is widely acknowledged that the terms are fairly imprecise, and can be stigmatizing, there are also attempts to combat this by defining them more rigorously and explaining them more clearly. And after all, so the argument goes, there has to be some way of categorizing people's distress, even if it is not perfect. Why not this one?

This chapter will explore the implications of diagnosis being the Holy Grail of psychiatry, and the key to its legitimization (Kovel, 1980). Some of the purposes of diagnosis and theory underpinning the use of medical diagnosis will be explored, highlighting the crucial role that the latter plays in psychiatry's claim to be a legitimate branch of medicine. It will be argued that theoretical justification for the diagnostic system is entirely lacking, with far-reaching consequences for psychiatry as it is currently conceived and practised. Indeed, as Brown (1990) states, 'any critique of diagnosis *is* the critique of psychiatry'. The largely destructive impact of diagnosis on service users will then be explored. The chapter concludes by outlining a number of alternatives to diagnosis, which are more valid and more useful.

The purposes of diagnosis

In general medicine, diagnosis is the essential first step towards prescribing the correct medical treatment. Diagnosis ideally also serves the following purposes, although they are not fulfilled in every case:

- It provides information and in some cases relief for patients and their carers, who want to know what condition they are suffering from.

- It enables predictions to be made about outcome, or prognosis.

- It enables professionals to communicate with each other in making their referrals, recommendations and treatment decisions.

- It provides a basis for research. We cannot research into a condition unless we have made some (provisional, at least) decision about how to define it and what name to give it.

- It informs us about aetiology, or causes, based on the research findings.

- It gives patients and carers access to services, benefits, support groups and so on.

How well does psychiatric diagnosis actually fulfil the purposes summarized above? Arguably, not very well. Although patients generally must have a label to access services, claim benefits and so on, there is a fairly loose relationship between diagnosis and medication regime in psychiatry, with most patients being tried on most drugs at some point during their career. Equally, it is hard to make precise predictions about outcome for most conditions (Ciompi, 1984). Despite confident talk about 'biochemical abnormalities', we have yet to identify any difference in brain chemistry that reliably correlates with mental distress – which in itself would be a long way from proving a causal link. Nor do we have firm evidence for claims about 'genetic vulnerabilities' (for a summary of the arguments see Johnstone, 2006a.) While it can be a relief to be given a diagnosis, it can also be experienced as shameful and stigmatizing. In addition, diagnostic practice varies so widely that it is hard to be certain that clinicians mean the same thing even if they use the same label (Kirk and Kutchins, 1994). There are obvious implications for research, which is bound to produce inconclusive and conflicting findings if it is not based on valid concepts in the first place.

All of these functions are very important, even if unfulfilled – and yet they are not the most crucial purpose that diagnosis serves for psychiatry. To appreciate this, we need to understand the implications of seeing psychiatry as a branch of medicine – in other words, as one of the natural sciences like biology, physics and chemistry (Ingleby, 1981). Any science needs to be based on a reliable and valid categorization of its basic units – whether these are atoms, chemicals or diseases – in order to develop testable hypotheses and hence the general laws that constitute a body of scientific knowledge. Without this basic classification system, none of the rest is possible. For example, if a precise and objective definition of an atom cannot be agreed upon, or of the different types of atom, there is no possibility of making hypotheses about what happens when they interact, and there would be no foundation for the science of chemistry. The equivalent in medicine is being able to define and classify types of illness, so that hypotheses about prognosis, aetiology, treatments and so on can be tested. As Kovel (1980) puts it, 'The medical model demands classification of its monads [i.e. units] along the order of somatic medical disease or any other set of physical objects. If this cannot be accomplished, then the whole model breaks down and scientific thinking is discarded.'

The absence of a reliable and valid classification system would, therefore, mean that psychiatry becomes 'something very hard to justify or defend – a medical speciality that does not treat medical illnesses' (Breggin, 1993). A moment's thought will demonstrate the far-reaching implications for psychiatry as it is currently practised, including the use of medical language (symptom, illness, patient, treatment, remission, prognosis, etc.); the typical settings (hospitals, wards, clinics); the medical training of key professionals (nurses and doctors); and the basic interventions (medication, ECT). All of these taken-for-granted aspects of psychiatry would be challenged by a threat to its diagnostic system and hence to its current status as a branch of medical science.

In order to examine these arguments more closely, there is a need to be clear about what exactly is meant by medical diagnosis, and how and why the biomedical model has come to play such a crucial part in Western models of psychiatry.

Diagnosis in context

Historical perspective

The founding father of the biomedical model of psychiatry was the German psychiatrist Emil Kraepelin, who, in 1887, produced the very first attempt to classify mental distress in medical terms (Bentall, 2003). After extensive research, he came to believe that the more severe psychiatric conditions essentially fell into three groups: dementia praecox; manic depression (now generally called 'bipolar disorder'); and paranoia. He believed, with no evidence, that the 'symptoms' associated with these conditions were manifestations of an underlying brain disease. Eugen Bleuler subsequently renamed the first category 'schizophrenia', and developed descriptions of the various subtypes of the condition. Karl Jaspers, another German psychiatrist, was responsible for elaborating the central assumption behind the diagnosis of psychosis, i.e. that the symptoms are *not understandable* within the context of the patient's life. Finally, Kurt Scheider described the so-called 'first-rank symptoms' of schizophrenia that still form the basis of today's diagnostic manuals, again with the emphasis on form, not content, of the delusions, hallucinations and so on. Together, these men established and elaborated the biomedical assumptions on which psychiatric diagnosis, and hence the whole field of psychiatry, is still based today (Bentall, 2003).

What is meant by medical diagnosis?

Boyle (1999) has helpfully summarized the process of developing and applying a medical diagnosis as follows:

> Firstly, the clinician or researcher must identify a pattern of *symptoms*, which are the complaints that commonly bring people to their doctor, such as nausea, pain and tiredness. Since these are largely subjective, and have many possible causes, a particular diagnosis can only be confirmed by the consistent association of this pattern with *signs*, such as measures of blood cell counts, abnormalities that show up on X rays and so on. Signs are objectively verifiable by others and can be compared with a norm, such as the expected cell count. The reliable association of certain clusters of symptoms with certain signs, where it is assumed that the sign precedes the symptoms, allows us to create a concept (commonly referred to as a diagnosis) such as 'diabetes' or 'arthritis'. This concept then becomes the basis for further research and refinement.

What are the differences between diagnosis in general medicine and in psychiatry?

Some of the DSM criteria for diagnosing schizophrenia are listed below (APA, 2000):

- Flat or grossly inappropriate affect.

- Digressive, vague, over-elaborate or circumstantial speech.

- Unusual perceptual experiences.

- Marked lack of initiative, interests or energy.

- Markedly peculiar behaviour (e.g. collecting garbage, talking to self in public, hoarding food).

- Marked impairment in personal hygiene and grooming.

- Odd beliefs or magical thinking, influencing behaviour and inconsistent with cultural norms.

Notoriously, there are no signs to confirm the presence or absence of a psychiatric disorder (with a few exceptions such as dementia); there is no blood test or X-ray to tell if someone really is suffering from psychosis. 'No one for whom Prozac has been prescribed has ever had their serotonin levels checked to see if they really are suffering from what the drug supposedly corrects' (Healy, 1998). While it is often stated as a fact that psychiatric disorders are caused by 'genetic vulnerability' or 'biochemical imbalances', there is actually no hard evidence at all to substantiate these theories. Readers are referred to other sources for more detailed discussion of these issues (Colbert, 2001; Joseph, 2004; Ross and Pam, 1995).

For these reasons, DSM provides lists of 'symptoms', not signs, as criteria for diagnosis. This makes the first problem with psychiatric diagnosis immediately obvious; without signs, there cannot be certainty that so-called psychiatric 'symptoms' are or are not evidence of a particular condition. Or indeed, whether these clusters of complaints are meaningful at all, rather than simply being a chance association. To use an analogy, psychiatrists are in the same position as a GP who, for some reason, has no access to standard medical tests, and who guesses that a patient's tiredness and weight loss are due to diabetes, but has no definite way of distinguishing this from cancer or simple lack of nutrition.

However, the problem goes deeper than this. It is important to note that DSM criteria such as those above are not, in fact, complaints about bodily functioning (pain, nausea and so on). They are examples of *beliefs, experiences and behaviours*. It is relatively simple, in principle, to work out how the body ought to be functioning and to draw up standards of normality with which signs can be compared: for example, checking to see if your blood pressure falls within an acceptable range. But there can be no such objective and universally agreed standards for deciding on 'normal' ways of feeling, thinking and behaving, because such judgements depend both on context (washing may be impossible if one is homeless) and culture (hearing voices may be acceptable in some societies.) There is no universal definition (or even a DSM attempt at one) of exactly how meticulous personal hygiene should be, or what is a reasonable level of initiative. Indeed, every single 'symptom', including the superficially more plausible ones (flat affect, unusual perceptual experiences) involves making an intrinsically subjective judgement. How flat does your affect have to be, and who decides this? How unusual is your perception, and where exactly do we draw the line that makes it so?

Nevertheless, such judgements are being made, or psychiatric diagnoses would not be used at all. This raises the important question of what kind of criteria are being used, if not the accepted medical one of the presence or absence of objective signs.

Interestingly, the answer is tacitly admitted within DSM itself in phrases such as 'bizarre beliefs...that the person's culture would regard as totally implausible' and 'odd beliefs...inconsistent with cultural norms'. It thus becomes clear that *the actual criteria for making a psychiatric diagnosis are social and cultural norms, which are dressed up as medical ones.*

This is even clearer in the case of the so-called 'personality disorders'. While these are not technically included under the category of 'mental illnesses', they do involve a psychiatrist's judgement of abnormality and possible referral to psychiatric services, with all the consequences that follow. Examples of the criteria for diagnosing them include (APA, 2000):

Conduct disorder: Unable to sustain consistent work behaviour; fails to conform to social norms with respect to lawful behaviour; abandonment of several jobs without realistic plans for others; has never sustained a totally monogamous relationship for more than one year; travelling from place to place without a rearranged job or clear goal; and so on.

Borderline personality disorder: A pattern of unstable and intense interpersonal relationships; markedly and persistently unstable self-image or sense of self; impulsivity in at least two areas that are potentially damaging, e.g. spending, eating disorders, reckless driving; inappropriate, intense anger.

There are recognizable individuals who fit these descriptions, and their behaviour may indeed be problematic; but note that in labelling them with a *disorder*, a value judgement is being made based on social/cultural norms ('this is not the way people should run their lives'), and not, as the diagnosis implies, a medical or scientific one.

One inevitable consequence is that those who are more culturally distant from the assumptions about 'normality' on which DSM is based are more likely to be given a psychiatric label, because diagnosis inevitably reflects and reinforces the norms of the white, western culture from which psychiatry has emerged. Research shows that this is indeed the case; e.g., Afro-Caribbeans living in the UK are up to twelve times more likely to be diagnosed with 'schizophrenia' (Fernando, 2002). These issues are explored further in chapter 3.

The process of turning personal and social problems into medical illnesses could be laughable when we read about cultures that are more distant in time and place; the 'drapetomania', or irresistible urge to run away from plantations that was said to afflict slaves in nineteenth-century America (Fernando, 2002), or the Soviet dissidents who were said to be suffering from 'paranoid delusions of reforming society'. It is more difficult to acknowledge that exactly the same processes occur today.

It follows from the above that psychiatrists are engaged in a kind of parody of orthodox medical practice: 'Psychiatrists behave *as if* they were studying bodily functioning and *as if* they had described patterns there, when in fact they are studying behaviour and have assumed – but not proved – that certain types of pattern *will be* found there' (Boyle, 2002).

It is important to be clear about the argument here. No one would deny that the people who present to mental health services often have serious problems; the issue is whether 'diagnosing' these problems as being caused by a medical 'illness' is a legitimate process. Equally, there is nothing intrinsically wrong with using subjectivity or what is sometimes called 'clinical judgement' to tell us about the person's difficulties. The problem arises when subjectivity is presented as objectivity, or to put it another way, social judgements are dressed up as medical ones. This has a number of practical consequences, both for psychiatry and for service users, which will be described below.

The consequences of psychiatric diagnosis for psychiatry

One of the most damaging consequences for psychiatry of basing diagnosis on social/cultural, not medical, norms is the consistent and inevitable failure to come up with a classification system that meets the basic scientific requirements of reliability and validity.

Reliability is the likelihood that different clinicians will agree upon a diagnosis in any given case. Any clinician will know that this is low; different psychiatrists have different diagnostic preferences, and patients commonly collect a range of diagnoses during their contact with mental health services. Research studies confirm that usage varies between different doctors, hospitals and countries. Even experienced clinicians, who have been given extra training in applying DSM criteria, only agree on a broad diagnostic category about half of the time (Kirk and Kutchins, 1994).

In an attempt to increase reliability, more and more diagnostic criteria have been added to DSM and ICD, creating hundreds of new disorders and subsections of disorders. There are two crucial problems with this tactic. The first is that the process is doomed to failure if the essentially subjective nature of the judgements remains; the extra criteria are no more scientific than the original ones.

The second problem is that while reliability is a necessary attribute of a scientific classification system, it is not on its own a sufficient one, because the categories also have to be shown to be valid. In other words, they need to reflect something meaningful in the real world. In biblical times, people were quite convinced that the mentally distressed had been taken over by evil spirits. In the seventeenth century there was widespread agreement on how to identify witches. The criteria used seemed to be very reliable, at least in most people's minds. This does not mean that 'witches' or evil spirits actually exist in the real world, as opposed to existing as a concept in our heads. It may seem very obvious, but it is hard to recognize that in confidently identifying 'schizophrenics' or 'personality disorders' exactly the same trap applies. These conditions cannot be seen, and they don't show up on tests, any more than evil spirits do, but somehow we are convinced that they are there – just like our seventeenth-century or biblical ancestors.

However, as will be apparent by now, the most serious consequence for psychiatry is the failure to support its claim to be a legitimate branch of medical science, with everything that follows from that.

The consequences of psychiatric diagnosis for the service user

In the absence of objective signs to confirm the presence of a biological disease process, psychiatry is left with a series of circular arguments. 'Why does this person hear voices?' 'Because they have schizophrenia.' 'How do you know they have schizophrenia?' 'Because they hear voices.' There is no exit from this circle via a sign such as a blood test for dopamine levels, or a brain scan for structural abnormalities.

The fact that this process is not scientifically meaningful does not, of course, imply that it is without consequences for the individual. Indeed, it is extremely powerful. As Rowe (1990) reminds us: 'In the final analysis, power is the right to have your definition of reality prevail over all other people's definition of reality.'

In the 'Purposes of diagnosis' list at the start of the chapter, it was noted that service users and their relatives naturally want to know what their condition is called. This can be a great relief ('Now we know what's wrong'), and a route to accessing services, benefits, self-help groups and so on. However, if such relief is based on the belief that the naming of the condition will lead to a specific and effective intervention, it may be short-lived. Moreover, relief is necessarily based on the assumption that the diagnosis itself is valid. The fact that service users and their carers have been seduced by the same rhetoric as most professionals does not mean their demands for a diagnosis should be agreed. If persuaded by the arguments in this chapter, this would be about as ethical as agreeing that the service user is possessed by evil spirits, or is a witch.

Even those who feel that psychiatric diagnosis has a role admit that it has undesirable practical consequences, including social isolation, difficulty in getting employment, housing and insurance, and gaining custody of or access to one's children after divorce. General discrimination because of the widespread stigma attached to mental health problems may also include being shouted at, threatened and physically attacked, harassed and intimidated at work (Barham and Hayward, 1995; Mehta and Farina, 1997; Read and Baker, 1996; Rogers, Pilgrim and Lacey, 1993; Sayce, 2000; and see Chapter 2).

All of the above is fairly widely acknowledged, and supported by a good deal of evidence. What is less explored is the *personal impact and meaning of psychiatric diagnosis*. Barham and Hayward (1995) vividly document the transition from personhood to patienthood that a psychiatric diagnosis instigates:

> I walked into (the psychiatrist's office) as Don and walked out a schizophrenic ... I remember feeling afraid, demoralised, evil.
>
> I am labelled for the rest of my life ... I think schizophrenia will always make me a second class citizen ... I haven't got a future.
>
> I'll never be able to erase the ink that's been put on me.
>
> (Honos-Webb and Leitner, 2001)
>
> The diagnosis becomes a burden ... you are an outcast in society. It took me years to feel OK about myself again.
>
> (Lindow, 1992)
>
> The killing of hope ... it almost feels like, well, your hands are tied, your cards laid and your fate set.
>
> (Horn, Johnstone and Brooke, 2007)

Honos-Webb and Leitner (2001) have explored how a DSM label can 'exacerbate symptoms and inhibit the healing process in therapy' by feeding into their core negative beliefs about themselves. Stereotyped public perceptions of the 'mentally ill' as weak, irresponsible and potentially violent are taken on as a central part of the person's identity, and the implication that they are abnormal, bad and crazy, and 'permanently stuck with this disorder', can induce a sense of alienation and despair that is profoundly anti-therapeutic.

As Honos-Webb and Leitner have argued, psychiatric diagnosis carries a number of powerful and damaging meta-messages, in addition to the stigma of the label itself (Johnstone, 2000):

Sick role: The common cultural understanding of being diagnosed as ill ('schizophrenic' or 'psychotic', etc.) is that you are not responsible for your condition, and need to rely on expert help to get better. While this may be true for cancer or pneumonia, it is generally not helpful for people going through a mental health crisis to be tacitly encouraged to give over responsibility for their recovery to the professionals, and wait for the pills to cure them. For their part, the professionals will quickly become frustrated with people who do not seem to be helping themselves, without quite appreciating the part that diagnosis plays in inviting them into this role. This sets the scene for the damaging game known as:

The rescue game: Since emotional breakdowns require people to take an active part in their own recovery, they do not get better from within the sick role, leading to a tendency for staff to *Persecute* (get frustrated with) them for their *Victim* position, in a gradual but predictable switch from pity to blame. Initially seen as having no responsibility (because they cannot help being 'psychotic' or whatever), service users are subsequently viewed as having complete responsibility for their feelings and behaviour; they are 'unmotivated' or 'enjoy being ill' or 'don't really want to change.' Service users in turn can get angry with staff and find various ways of *Persecuting* them back, many of which, such as being aggressive/demanding or helpless/dependent, are permitted within the cultural meaning of what it is to be 'mentally ill'. Each side take turns to adopt the positions of *Rescuer*, *Persecutor* and *Victim*, which is a no-win situation for everyone. (Karpman, 1968).

The treatment barrier: The process of redefining relationship problems as medical ones has been described in some classic papers by Scott (1973a, 1973b) as creating a 'treatment barrier'. When all the difficulties have been officially located within one person ('the doctor says he has a mental illness'), and then sealed off behind a diagnostic label, it is extremely hard for staff to do any work on couple or family dynamics at any later stage, however important a part they play. The scene is set for the identified person to embark on a lifelong career within the psychiatric system, with relationship and social issues not only unaddressed but concealed and reinforced. The cost, to staff and service users, is extremely high.

Perhaps the most damaging consequence of diagnosis, underpinning all the other factors, is *the loss of personal meaning*. This is intrinsic to the biomedical assumptions that date all the way back to Kraepelin. If hearing voices, or being low in mood, or intensely anxious, or fearing that you are being poisoned by your relatives, are diagnosed as the 'symptoms' of an 'illness', there is no more reason for professionals to enquire into them than into the meaning of a rash, or the content of delirious speech in a fever. Factors such as past abuse, neglect and trauma will be noted as part of the psychiatric history and probably never discussed again, while numerous variations on medication to treat the 'illness' are tried. As a result, patients can spend years rotating in and out of hospital without anyone sitting down and trying to help them make sense of their distress in terms that are personally meaningful to them. This is by far the biggest source of service-user dissatisfaction: 'Respondents saw their difficulties as meaningful in the context of their life experiences...Being treated in a medicalised way, as if they had physical illnesses, formed the basis of negative evaluations and complaints on the part of most service users in every aspect of their management' (Rogers, Pilgrim and Lacey, 1993). In other words, 'the professional discourse and the lay discourse about personal distress are incompatible'. Service users typically see themselves as having broken down for *reasons* which remain largely unaddressed within a model that defines them as suffering from *illnesses.*

In summary, the process of redefining service users' psychological and social problems as symptoms of an illness is not simply unscientific and unjustified by evidence. It is an immensely powerful act, which has profoundly damaging implications for the individual's identity, relationships, place in the community, ability to benefit from therapy, employment, health and future. In Barham and Hayward's (1995) words, 'an impoverished conception of what (they) can reasonably do and hope for – of (their) significance and value – have been brought to merge in a painful experience of exclusion and worthlessness'. Short-term relief and access to services are outweighed by the long-term disadvantages of:

- removing meaning
- obscuring relationship and social contexts
- Individualizing problems
- removing responsibility ('sick role')
- disempowering and stigmatizing
- keeping relationships stuck ('treatment barrier')
- medical consequences (medication)
- social/practical consequences (unemployment, discrimination, etc.).

Taking all this into account, it is not surprising that many service users experience being given a diagnosis of mental illness as one of the most damaging aspects of their contact with the services. It is also unsurprising to find that recovery, if it does happen, seems to be facilitated by being able to reject your diagnosis (Warner, 2004). A key figure in the Recovery Movement describes this turning point: 'In the early 1980s I was diagnosed as schizophrenic...In 1993 I gave up being schizophrenic and decided to be Ron Coleman.'

Of course, this is not easy. As Coleman says, this 'means taking back responsibility for yourself, it means that you can no longer blame your illness for your actions...but more important, it means that you stop being a victim of your experience and start being the owner of your experience' (Coleman, 1999).

International perspectives

Research and debate about diagnosis from an international perspective tends to fall into three main areas:

* Patterns of diagnosis in minority ethnic groups, as discussed briefly above (such as Littlewood and Lipsedge, 1997).

* So-called 'culture-bound syndromes', which often sound exotic to westerners, such as the diagnosis of 'windigo' in Algonquin Indians who develop a fear that they have been bewitched, or *taijin kyofusho* in Japan, in which sufferers have a deep fear of offending or hurting others. These are listed in the appendix to DSM-IV.

* Cross-cultural research looking at, for example, the incidence of 'schizophrenia' in the developing world (such as Warner, 2004).

Transcultural psychiatrists like Littlewood and Lipsedge (1997) have argued that psychiatric diagnosis needs to be carried out with especial care with members of minority ethnic groups, so that understandable reactions to cultural conflicts and contexts are not misdiagnosed as a 'mental illness'. They do not, however, question the validity of the diagnostic process itself.

A more radical critique comes from Fernando (2002), who argues strongly that since all psychiatric diagnosis is inherently laden with western values and assumptions, it simply cannot be applied or understood in a non-western culture. Western medicine, for example, assumes a split between mind and body that is completely absent in traditional African, Asian and Native American worldviews. Such cultures have no exact equivalent to our diagnostic practices, and may see what is defined as psychiatric disorders in religious, spiritual, philosophical or ethical terms instead. To seek to impose models of medicine on their experiences is to fall into the racist assumption that ones worldview is superior because it is more 'true'. This can be described as a form of 'psychiatric imperialism'; more subtle, but no less damaging, than more overt forms of colonialism.

Incorporating some non-western perspectives would mean that psychiatry 'would need to give up its outdated model of the individualised person (and) rewrite its diagnostic systems in line with a holistic understanding that addresses the connectedness between people, the environment and the cosmos'. However, 'if such changes occur, it may be difficult to recognise the result as "psychiatry" anyway' (Fernando, 2002).

In fact, although all societies seem to recognize some sort of 'madness', Fernando does not believe that a universal language about what is called mental illness is possible, since each model would only be valid within its own culture. He does, however, have a number of suggestions for a truly multicultural psychiatry in the West, which incorporates many of the features that service users of all ethnic backgrounds are campaigning for. This includes 'diagnosis... being superseded in importance by an understanding of the individual in the context of family and society ... Psychiatrists would move away from seeing "symptoms" such as hallucinations as "disorders" ... towards seeing them as experiences with meaning and significance' (Fernando, 2003).

Future vision: responses to the above

The psychiatric profession has, of course, been aware of the controversy around diagnosis at least since the 1960s, when it surfaced in the widely read critiques of R.D. Laing, Thomas Szasz and others. Laing's key contention was that 'schizophrenia' is not a valid category, but denotes behaviours that can be seen as a meaningful and understandable response to damaging family relationships (Laing, 1960; Laing and Esterson, 1964). Szasz saw the concept of 'mental illness' as meaningless, and attacked the continuing search for brain lesions to justify drugging and incarcerating people whom we find disturbing (Szasz, 1976). This controversy has not gone away. For example, one of the open debates in the Maudsley series in 2003 was on the topic 'Does schizophrenia exist?' – a question that resulted, after a show of hands at the end, in a draw (Van Os and McKenna, 2003).

One typical response to critiques of psychiatric diagnosis is, 'You have to categorise people's conditions somehow.' This leads to attempts to lessen some of its disadvantages; for example, the Royal College of Psychiatry's anti-stigma campaign 'Changing minds: Every family in the land' (Cowan and Hart, 1998). As a variation on this theme, it is sometimes suggested that new versions of particularly stigmatizing labels should be introduced (e.g. 'dopamine dysregulation disorder' for 'schizophrenia'; Murray, 2006).

The problem with this kind of response is that it does not seem to work. A review article by Read *et al.* (2006) found that despite many such campaigns across the western world over the years, 'the public, including service users and carers ... continue to prefer psychosocial explanations and treatments'. Moreover, adopting beliefs about biological causation is consistently related to greater, not less, prejudice, fear and desire for distance (Read *et al.*, 2006).

Another strategy is to replace a diagnosis that seems less credible with another one. For example, the term 'shell-shock' was introduced in the First World War when it became increasingly implausible to diagnose the vast number of traumatized soldiers as suffering from a mass outbreak of psychosis. The exponential growth in the number of people diagnosed with 'borderline personality disorder' and 'bipolar disorder' is perhaps another instance of moving the goalposts, which may temporarily silence those who dislike certain labels. However, it is no answer to the fundamental problems inherent in the diagnostic process itself.

There is a current trend to replace 'schizophrenia' with the less precise and perhaps less alarming general term 'psychosis'. Not all service users are convinced that this is much of an improvement. However, a moment's thought will show that such a broad category implies even greater problems of reliability and validity, without fully avoiding biomedical assumptions and all the problems therein.

More radical alternatives

The recently established 'Campaign to abolish the schizophrenia label' (www.asylumonline.net) has quickly inspired affiliated groups across the UK and in several other countries. Its supporters argue that 'The concept of schizophrenia is unscientific and has outlived any usefulness it may once have claimed'; and, moreover, that 'A single word can ruin a life as surely as any bullet, and schizophrenia is just such a word.' It seems as if the time may be ripe for a fundamental rethinking of psychiatric diagnosis.

Real alternatives to psychiatric diagnosis need to avoid the trap of assuming that the scientific categorization of mental distress is possible or necessary at all. It goes without saying that there have to be ways of understanding and making sense of the world through grouping things together – starting as an infant with 'mother' versus 'other people' and developing into highly sophisticated ways of organizing experiences. However, there is generally no expectation or need for such categories to meet scientific standards of reliability and validity. Nor is this necessary in the field of mental health if we are dealing with *human distress*, rather than *medical illnesses*. Why should it be expected to fall into neat clusters with precise characteristics? And of course, all the research confirms that it doesn't (Boyle, 2002). If clinicians see themselves, as service users tell us they see themselves (wrestling with a messy, complex mixture of traumatic life events, relationship conflicts and adverse social circumstances), then the question needing to be asked is not 'What kind of illness is this?' but 'What kind of problem is this?' And one possible answer to this is not a *diagnosis* but a *formulation*.

What is a formulation?

A formulation can be defined as 'a hypothesis about a person's difficulties, which draws from psychological theory' (Johnstone and Dallos, 2006). In other words, it is an individual summary, developed collaboratively with the service user, which looks at all aspects of a person's life in order to try and explain how and why their problems arose, and what interventions, if any, will be useful. Formulations can best be understood as hypotheses to be tested (Butler, 1998). All formulations are based on the assumption that ... at some level it all makes sense (Butler, 1998). In other words, formulations give a central role to the exploration of *personal meaning*. This, of course, is the polar opposite to the assumptions inherited from Kraepelin, Bleuler, Jaspers and Schneider (see table 1.1).

Here is a hypothetical example:

Diagnostic approach. Present state examination: Mrs Smith was born to a depressed mother and was sexually abused by her father. She did badly at school, and her parents separated when she was 10. She started cutting herself as a teenager. She had relationships with a number of abusive men before getting married and having two children. After the second birth, she started hearing voices which accused her of wanting to harm her children. She became depressed and unable to care for her children, and was admitted to hospital and given a diagnosis of schizo-affective disorder. *Main intervention*: neuroleptics.

Formulation approach. Initial interview: Since her mother was not able to care for her properly, Jane never developed a secure sense of herself or of her own

Table 1.1 Diagnosis versus formulation

Diagnosis	Formulation
Removes meaning	Seeks meaning
Removes responsibility ('sick role')	Promotes responsibility
Obscures social contexts	Includes social contexts
Individualizes	Includes relationships
Keeps relationships stuck ('treatment barrier')	Looks at relationship change
Disempowers	Is collaborative
Stigmatizes	Is non-stigmatizing
Is hard to remove	Is always open to revision
Has medical consequences (medication, etc.)	Is non-medical
Has social consequences	Has no social consequences

self-worth. This was compounded by the abuse she was subjected to, which left her with profound feelings of anger, worthlessness and guilt. She takes this out on herself in the form of self-injury, finding temporary relief but in the long run increasing her despair. Desperate for love and security, but not feeling she deserved a caring relationship, she became involved with a number of unsuitable partners. Each relationship confirmed her feelings of rejection and failure when it ended. She loves her children but often finds their emotional needs overwhelming, having so many unmet needs herself. Her voices may represent this dilemma, as well as her unresolved guilt about her part in the abuse. *Intervention*: establish a trusting relationship in which she can express her feelings, explore the effects of the abuse, come to accept herself and find alternatives to self-harm; arrange help with parenting skills and childcare; join a Hearing Voices group to develop coping strategies for the voices; review and revise the formulation with her as necessary.

A similar approach is used in the 'Need-adapted' model from Finland, based on systemic and psychodynamic theories which 'make diagnosis problematic ... [and] of limited use ... The integrated and need-adapted approach is founded on being problem-oriented' (Alanen *et al.*, 2002). In practice this means that categories such as 'identity crisis' and 'separation crisis', which could be seen as broad-level formulations, are used in preference to terms like 'schizophrenia'. Another variation is found in the Bradford Home Treatment team, where the service 'attempts to work with a "needs-led" approach and does not ... seek to diagnose the service user's problems in a medical way' (Bracken and Thomas, 2002). Finally, in Japan, the term for 'mind-split disease', equivalent to our 'schizophrenia', has been replaced, after campaigning by service users and carers, by 'integration disorder', defined as 'a syndrome ... whose etiology and physiology are not yet firmly established' (Sato, 2006). The Hearing Voices Network, a user-led organization that views hearing voices as a variation of normal human experience rather than the manifestation of a diseases process, is committed to creating 'an acceptance that hearing voices is a valid experience for which there are many possible explanations … we accept the explanation of each voice hearer' (www.hearing-voices.org).

It would be naïve to suggest that a formulation-based approach is an answer to all the problems inherent in psychiatric diagnosis (Boyle, 2001; Johnstone, 2006b). However, it does in principle offer a way of reintroducing *personal meaning, personal responsibility, personal relationships* and *social contexts* into mental health work, while avoiding the propensity of diagnosis to individual-ize problems, stigmatize the individual, and encourage service users to rely on external medical solutions (Johnstone, 2006b). As such, it can be seen as a genuine alternative to (not simply an addition to) psychiatric diagnosis (Pilgrim, 2000).

Summary

Psychiatric diagnosis is flawed in theory and damaging in practice, and a significant number of professionals and service users argue for it to be aban-doned. There are realistic and practical alternatives, which are already being implemented in some services. The full implications for the practice of psychiatry have yet to be worked through.

EDITORS' QUESTIONS

Issues of difference

- A diagnosis such as borderline personality disorder is much more often ascribed to women. Why might this be?

- Why do you think homosexuality was once a psychiatric disorder?

- In what ways might cultural differences influence whether someone is given a psychiatric diagnosis?

Relevance to practice

- A service user has been given a diagnosis and you disagree with the use of diagnosis. What can you do?

- In what way can ignorance of the limitations of diagnoses hinder practice?

- What alternatives would you consider to diagnosis?

Investigate

- What are the problems with psychiatric diagnoses?

- What are the differences between a diagnostic and formulation approach?

- How can you help reduce the impact for the person labelled with a psychiatric diagnosis?

Suggested further reading

Boyle, M. (2002) *Schizophrenia: A Scientific Delusion?* (2nd edn). London and New York: Routledge.

Johnstone, L. (2000) *Users and Abusers of Psychiatry: A Critical Look at Psychiatric Practice* (2nd edn). London and Philadelphia: Routledge.

References

Alanen, Y.O., Lehtinen, V., Lehtinen, K., Aaltonen, J., and Rakkolainen, V. (2002) The Finnish integrated model for early treatment of schizophrenia and related psychoses. In B. Martindale, A. Bateman, M. Crowe, and F. Margison (eds) *Psychosis: Psychological Approaches and their Treatment*. London: Gaskell.

APA (2000) *Diagnostic and Statistical Manual of Mental Disorders* (4th edn), *DSM-IV-TR*. Washington, DC: American Psychiatric Association.

Barham, P. and Hayward, R. (1995) *Re-locating Madness: From the Mental Patient to the Person*. London: Free Association Books.

Bentall, R. (2003) *Madness Explained: Psychosis and Human Nature*. London: Penguin.

Boyle, M. (1999) Diagnosis. In C. Newnes, G. Holmes, and C. Dunn (eds) *This Is Madness: A Critical Look at Psychiatry and the Future of the Mental Health Services*. Ross-on-Wye: PCCS Books.

Boyle, M. (2001) Abandoning diagnosis and (cautiously) adopting formulation. Paper presented at the British Psychological Society Centenary Conference, Glasgow.

Boyle, M. (2002) *Schizophrenia: A Scientific Delusion?* (2nd edn). London and New York: Routledge.

Bracken, P. and Thomas, P. (2002) Time to move beyond the mind–body split. *British Medical Journal*, **325**: 1433–4.

Breggin, P. (1993) *Toxic Psychiatry*. London: Fontana.

Brown, P. (1990) The name game: towards a sociology of diagnosis. *Journal of Mind and Behaviour*, **11**: 385–406.

Butler, G. (1998) Clinical formulation. In A.S. Bellack and M. Hersen (eds) *Comprehensive Clinical Psychology*. Oxford: Pergamon.

Ciompi, L. (1984) Is there really a schizophrenia? The long-term course of psychotic phenomena, *British Journal of Psychiatry*, **145**: 636–40.

Colbert, T. (2001) *Rape of the Soul: How the Chemical Imbalance Model of Modern Psychiatry Has Failed Its Patients*. Tustin, CA: Kevco.

Coleman, R. (1999) Hearing voices and the politics of oppression. In C. Newnes, G. Holmes and C. Dunn (eds) *This Is Madness: A Critical Look at Psychiatry and the Future of the Mental Health Services*. Ross-on-Wye, PCCS Books.

Cowan, L. and Hart, D. (1998) Changing minds: every family in the land: a new challenge for the future (editorial). *Psychiatric Bulletin*, **22**: 593–4.

Fernando, S. (2002) *Mental Health, Race and Culture* (2nd edn). Basingstoke and New York: Palgrave Macmillan.

Fernando, S. (2003) *Cultural Diversity, Mental Health and Psychiatry: the Struggle against Racism*, Hove, New York: Brunner-Routledge.

Healy, D. (1998) Gloomy days and sunshine pills. *Openmind*, **90**: 8–9.

Honos-Webb, L. and Leitner, L.M. (2001) How using the DSM causes damage: a client's report. *Journal of Humanistic Psychology*, **41**: 4, 36–56.

Horn, N., Johnstone, L., and Brooke, S. (2007) Some service user perspectives on the diagnosis of Borderline Personality Disorder. *Journal of Mental Health*, **16**(2): 255–69.

Ingleby, D. (1981) Understanding 'mental illness'. In D. Ingleby (ed.) *Critical Psychiatry: The Politics of Mental Health*. Harmondsworth: Penguin.

Johnstone, L. (2000) *Users and Abusers of Psychiatry: A Critical Look at Psychiatric Practice* (2nd edn). London and Philadelphia: Routledge.

Johnstone, L. (2006a) The limits of biomedical models of distress. In D. Double (ed.) *Critical Psychiatry: The Limits of Madness*. London: Palgrave Macmillan.

Johnstone, L. (2006b) Controversies and debates in formulation. In L. Johnstone and R. Dallos (eds) *Formulation in Psychology and Psychotherapy: Making Sense of People's Problems*. London, New York: Routledge.

Johnstone, L. and Dallos, R. (2006) Introduction to formulation. In L. Johnstone and R. Dallos (eds) *Formulation in Psychology and Psychotherapy: Making Sense of People's Problems*, London, New York: Routledge.

Joseph, J. (2004) *The Gene Illusion: Genetic Research in Psychiatry and Psychology under the Microscope*, Ross-on-Wye: PCCS Books.

Karpman, S.B. (1968) Script drama analysis. *Transactional Analysis Bulletin*, 7(26), 39–43.

Kirk, S. and Kutchins, H. (1994) The myth of the reliability of DSM. *Journal of Mind and Behaviour*, 15(1–2): 71–86.

Kovel, J. (1980) The American mental health industry. In D. Ingleby (ed.) *Critical Psychiatry: The Politics of Mental Health*. Harmondsworth: Penguin.

Laing, R.D. (1960) *The Divided Self.* London: Tavistock.

Laing, R.D. and Esterson, A. (1964) *Sanity, Madness and the Family*. London: Tavistock.

Lindow, V. (1992) A service user's view. In H. Wright and M. Goddey (eds) *Mental Health Nursing: From First Principles to Professional Practice*. London: Chapman & Hall.

Littlewood, R. and Lipsedge, M. (1997) *Aliens and Alienists: Ethnic Minorities and Psychiatry* (3rd edn). London and New York: Routledge.

Mehta, S. and Farina, A. (1997) Is being 'sick' really better? Effect of the disease view of mental disorder on stigma. *Journal of Social and Clinical Psychology*, 16(4): 405–19.

Murray, R (2006) quoted on Campaign for the Abolition of the Schizophrenia website: http://www.asylumonline.net [accessed 16/09/2007].

Pilgrim, D. (2000) Psychiatric diagnosis: more questions than answers. *The Psychologist*, 13(6): 302–5.

Read, J. and Baker, S. (1996) *Not Just Sticks and Stones: A Survey of Stigma, Taboos and Discrimination Experienced by People with Mental Health Problems*. London: MIND.

Read, J., Haslam, N., Sayce, L. and Davies, E. (2006) Prejudice and schizophrenia: a review of the 'mental illness is an illness like any other' approach. *Acta Psychiatrica Scandinavica*, 114: 303–18.

Rogers, A., Pilgrim, D., and Lacey, R. (1993) *Experiencing Psychiatry: Users' Views of Services*. London: Macmillan.

Ross, C.A. and Pam, A. (1995) *Pseudoscience in Biological Psychiatry: Blaming the Body*. New York: Wiley.

Rowe, D. (1990) Introduction. In J. Masson, *Against Therapy*. London: Fontana.

Sato, M (2006) Re-naming schizophrenia: a Japanese perspective. *World Psychiatry*, 5(1): 53–5.

Sayce, L. (2000) *From Psychiatric Patient to Citizen: Overcoming Discrimination and Social Exclusion*. London: Palgrave Macmillan.

Scott, R.D. (1973a) The treatment barrier: part 1. *British Journal of Medical Psychology*, 46: 45–55.

Scott, R.D. (1973b) The treatment barrier: part 2. *British Journal of Medical Psychology*, 46: 57–67.

Szasz, T. (1976) Schizophrenia: the sacred symbol of psychiatry. *British Journal of Psychiatry*, **129**: 308–16.

van Os, J. and McKenna, P. (2003) *Does Schizophrenia Exist?* Maudsley Discussion Paper no. 12. London: Institute of Psychiatry Media Support Unit.

Warner, R. (2004) *Recovery from Schizophrenia: Psychiatry and Political Economy* (3rd edn). Hove and New York: Brunner-Routledge.

Socioeconomic Disadvantage

David Pilgrim and Anne Rogers

BRIEF CHAPTER OUTLINE

The following chapter explores the concept that social judgements disvalue people with mental health problems and therefore saturate mental health status. This is achieved by answering a set of questions that draw mainly from social psychiatry and medical sociology. The questions are:

▨ What is the link between labour-market position and mental health?

▨ What is the impact of 'mental health services' on social exclusion?

▨ What intergenerational and intragenerational effects are evident?

▨ What types of capital affect mental health?

▨ What is the relationship between people and neighbourhoods?

▨ How coherent is professional knowledge for our understanding of mental health in its social context?

Introduction

For anyone working with or researching people with mental health problems, it is fairly evident that they are often poor. It is also clear that the forms of oppression and disadvantage typically attending poverty, such as poor education, low pay or unemployment, poor neighbourhoods and poor living conditions, enhance neither physical nor mental health (Fryers, Melzer and Jenkins, 2000; Rogers and Pilgrim, 2003). Class position predicts both morbidity in its broadest sense and longevity in its specific sense. Not only do the poor consistently die younger, but this pattern of early death is amplified in poor people who also have a psychiatric diagnosis (Knapp, 2001). Also, whatever the original causes of mental health problems, the negative social consequences of being in contact with specialist services and receiving a psychiatric diagnosis are considerable. The stigma and personal invalidation this brings are then joined by a good chance of exclusion from the labour market (Alexander and Link, 2003; Sayce, 2000).

But to limit this chapter to these matters about psychiatric patienthood alone would miss many important nuances of understanding. For example, most people with mental health problems are not psychiatric patients; they never leave primary medical care. Some do not even consult their general practitioner; community surveys detect a clinical iceberg of symptoms in people who are not patients. This is true, whether we examine the symptoms of misery ('common mental disorders') or madness ('serious and enduring mental illness') (Delespaul, de Vries and van Os, 2002; Tien, 1991; van Os *et al.*, 2000).

Of those who do present to general practitioners, a high proportion arguably have a primary disability (usually codified medically as 'depression' or work related 'stress'), which is the reason often voluntarily agreed between patient and doctor to remove the former for some period of time from the labour market. This suggests that we need to have an eye on mental health as a *reason* for socioeconomic disadvantage, as well as seeking evidence for discrimination and exclusion, once a diagnosis has occurred.

Indeed, circular relationships, rather than linear ones, capture the relationship between the social and the mental health of persons and render older arguments about social stress and downward social drift as futile. The latter debate, which focused on psychosis, was an argument about which comes first, poverty or madness. Social drift arguments were strongly linked to claims about genetic vulnerability. However, even if downward drift were evident, psychiatric disability could accrue historically from environmental factors and so the social would still be implicated.

Logically and empirically, individual vulnerability is much more than genetic. The relevance of social stress mediated by family and other intimate networks could be historical ('aetiological factors'), current ('proximate triggers') or prospective ('maintenance factors'). And diagnosis is a social negotiation (not a self-evident fact waiting to be discovered). Some people have always been mad or miserable, but only modern patients can suffer from 'schizophrenia' or 'depression'. And these states occur more in some social groups than others. Social judgements then disvalue people with mental health problems.

Thus, the social saturates mental health status. This saturation is explored below in relation to the chapter topic via a set of questions. In answering these, sources are drawn from social psychiatry and medical sociology. Finally, we reflect on the coherence of this mixture of sources.

What is the link between labour-market position and mental health?

The social and environmental factors impinging on mental health are multiple. Later the chapter deals with neighbourhood effects. In this section the evidence about a commonly associated topic – employment – is summarized by a series of bullet points.

- *The social context of unemployment is crucial.* This point is about the labour market in, rather than as part of, a social context. Put simply, labour-market effects are reliant on the presence or absence of state-provided income maintenance and on the circumstances in which a person becomes unemployed. In most developed countries unemployed people have the safety net of welfare payments. In Britain these include unemployment and invalidity benefits. These ensure that poverty is relative, not absolute, as resources are made available to sustain food and shelter. In some developing countries this safety net is absent. For example, Patel (2001) notes that in India during the mid-1990s many low-paid bonded farmers lost everything when the monsoon destroyed their crops. They were immediately propelled into absolute poverty and suicide levels dramatically increased. In the other direction, some forms of unemployment may be linked to financial and social advantages (for example, when receiving a good retirement package or when inheriting wealth). This is not to argue that unemployment does not affect mental health in developed countries, but it does lead to the next, counter-intuitive, point.

- *Poor employment, not unemployment, has the largest detrimental impact on mental health.* The worst mental health is found not in unemployed people but in those on low pay and with poor task control, on short-term contracts or in informal work roles – sometimes called 'inadequate employment' (Dooley, Prause and Ham-Rowbottom, 2000; Ludermir and Lewis, 2003). The best mental health is found in higher wage earners with good task control and permanent contracts. Poor task control and conflict with managers are associated with neurotic distress in workers (Andrea *et al.*, 2004). This suggests that while unemployment has many stressors, which negatively affect morale and increase the risk of neurotic symptoms (Jenkins *et al.*, 2003), work brings with it its own peculiar and predictable stress, as well as status, structured daily activity and, of course, earnings. Moreover, within the workforce, some occupations are at greater risk than others of mental health problems (Wilhelm *et al.*, 2004).

- *Unemployment and low pay have direct and indirect effects on mental health*; both ensure poverty and with this come both the environmental effects discussed later in relation to neighbourhood and the psychological effects of low status. In the case of becoming unemployed, these effects can be compounded by multiple losses (Fryer, 1995). For many, identity is bound up with work roles (loss of identity). For others, daily meanings are bound up with the routines of work (loss of daily structure). For some, being unemployed is a source of shame (loss of face). And for those whose income levels drop significantly, there is the direct impact of the loss of money. However, the latter applies less to those in the poverty trap. These people gain little or nothing by shifting from no pay to low pay. To offset losses of status, routine and buying power, unemployed people also have some opportunities (for leisure and rest) that are not available for people in insecure employment. Also, the unemployed person may potentially adapt to a secure identity outside the labour market, and life there can develop a degree of predictability. By contrast, the insecurely employed person can be in chronic fear of anticipated loss.

■ *Macro-economic effects are important.* Economic cycles create advantages and disadvantages to individuals (Kasl, Rodrigues and Lasch, 1998). For example, one generation of young people might encounter a period of growth and can access the labour market readily. The next generation may be less fortunate. Those in insecure employment will be buffered from its effects during times of full employment, but in more economically depressed times will be very vulnerable (Pearlin and Scaff, 1996).

Thus the relationship between the labour market and mental health is complex. This is not simply a matter of looking, stereotypically, for evidence that unemployment is bad for mental health. We now challenge another stereotype: that mental health services exist to improve mental health.

What is the impact of 'mental health services' on social exclusion?

The question is answered differently by different interest groups, which broadly fall into two camps. In the first are those who emphasize that people who are mentally disordered (whether this is codified as 'mental illness', 'personality disorder' or 'substance misuse') should have access to well-resourced professional services to ameliorate their problems. If those so afflicted are unaware of their needs (because they lack insight), then professionals have a duty of care to ensure treatment. This position, which is occupied by most mental health professionals and politicians and some charity groups, combines paternalism and scientism. The assumption is that there is a moral obligation to treat those who are psychologically different and that there is scientific evidence that this treatment is effective.

In the second group are critics of this orthodoxy who are anti-paternalistic and who privilege the right to be different. They also argue that evidence of effectiveness has to be set against the iatrogenic damage done to service recipients. This damage includes the direct impact of treatments (unwanted or 'side' effects) and the indirect impact of social stigma attending service contact and the receipt of a psychiatric diagnosis.

Given these different perspectives on the worthiness of specialist services, the latter can either be framed as a resource to be distributed equitably to those in need, or as part of the state apparatus to suppress residual deviance. As a consequence of these quite discrepant perspectives, services can either be viewed as a response to need or as a threat to well-being. If the first view is taken, then the arguments centre on the willingness of the state to provide adequate levels of funding for a full and competent mental health workforce. Put differently, patients not having access to these services are seen as suffering from a form of deprivation. If the second view is taken, a totally different construction becomes apparent. The challenge is not to access services but to avoid them or at least evade their iatrogenic impact. This entails people with mental health problems coping alone, seeking help from peers or accessing professional help, which is non-coercive and client-centred.

The first view has been the direction taken by psychiatric epidemiology. The latter has mapped out the incidence and prevalence on a range of diagnostic groups with a view to identifying the level of service availability implied for localities. X number of people 'with schizophrenia' implies Y number of beds, staff and money. With this view comes an ideology of benign paternalism – if these resources are not made available by the state, then patients are being disadvantaged and treated in a discriminatory way.

However, psychiatric epidemiology has not been commensurable with the second position (taken by most sociologists and some critical services users and professionals). This counter-view argues that service need to be understood as part of an apparatus of social control. Accordingly what is implied is not more, but less, access to statutory services and more, not fewer, alternatives to routine psychiatric care. During the twentieth century, what, in the UK, is now called 'mental health services' emerged from two quite separate projects about psychological deviance: one characterized by coercion and the other by voluntarism.

The first was the legacy of the Victorian lunacy policy. In the last Act in this phase, that of 1890, all patients entering asylums were certified and detained involuntarily. By the 1930 Mental Treatment Act, the possibility of 'voluntary boarders' emerged, but for many years only a minority of hospital residents were voluntary. By the 1960s, after the 1959 Mental Health Act, only a minority were officially recorded as 'formal' (coercively detained).

By the 1990s, with the large hospitals gone and small acute units with few beds now operating in localities, the ratio changed again, with the majority now being detained compulsorily. Post-1930, this ratio was imprecise because voluntary or 'informal' patients were subjected to the 'hidden section' of being pressured to enter and stay quietly, knowing that to do otherwise would lead to formal detention (Rogers, 1993; Szmuckler and Appelbaum, 2001). Thus the push and pull of the ratio of voluntary to involuntary residency in psychiatric beds has been a function of public policy about the asylum system and the more residual function of the acute unit. Both the large hospitals and the smaller acute units are explicitly about managing risky behaviour, though the former was in a position also to offer permanent accommodation. Psychiatric wards are rarely treatment centres to ameliorate distress or promote mental health (even though, misleadingly, they are often called 'mental health units').

Unlike most forms of health service, which confirm the 'inverse care law', of the poorest in the population being underrepresented in their access to care (Tudor-Hart, 1971), the opposite is true of psychiatric services. In the latter poor people are *overrepresented*. Accordingly, whatever the rhetorical gloss about 'treatment under the mental health act' psychiatric professionals working with inpatients have been agents of social control.

Coercive psychiatry *ipso facto* succeeds by socially excluding deviant individuals. Social exclusion is a sign of success – the psychiatric profession operates to regulate some behavioural manifestations of poverty – even if this success is not a matter of professional pride. Accordingly, the chance of coercive control increases with declining class position (Bindman *et al.*, 2002). Because of their role in amplifying social exclusion, it is not surprising that in countries where specialist services are less developed, we find that social inclusion and its positive impact on prognosis is evident (Warner, 1985). It is also not surprising that estimates of levels of unemployment in service users vary from 45 to 90 per cent internationally (Ruesch *et al.*, 2004). This is not to argue that service contact is the sole reason for high levels of unemployment, as community stigma and primary disability also play their part (Marwaha and Johnson, 2004), but it is to argue that service contact is a factor in maintaining rather than reversing social exclusion.

Turning to the second and voluntary face of psychiatry, poststructuralist writers have challenged the sociological consensus about coercive social control. Typical of this view is this succinct point from Miller and Rose (1988), 'We argue that it is more fruitful to consider the ways that regulatory systems have sought to promote subjectivity than document ways they have crushed it.' This allusion to the productive rather than repressive manifestation of power emerged in the main after the First World War. The psychiatric focus on madness did not disappear – it remained central – but it was joined by a fresh interest in neurosis.

Once the ambit of psychiatry and wider apparatus now called 'mental health services' expanded it was not just about coercive social control. Increasingly some of these services became true services – they were 'anxiously sought and gratefully received' (Ingleby, 1981). Whether the latter patients were treated medicinally or with new technologies of the self (the psychotherapies), the social management of psychological deviance could now be understood as a negotiated, not an imposed, order and as a set of discursive practices that both professionals and patients voluntarily inhabited (Rose, 1979, 1986, 1990).

This picture can largely be seen in primary care, where most mental health problems are medically codified and responded to, not in the statutory services. Statutory psychiatric services have now largely become psychosis services, with psychotherapy with its emphasis on voluntarism being firmly on their margins. But in primary care we find a shifting ratio of medicinal and psychological technical responses (anxiolytics, anti-depressants, cognitive behaviour therapy and counselling) to problems of living for those never seeing a psychiatrist or other specialist mental health worker.

And this division is important because it highlights that most people with mental health problems never enter the psychiatric system. The latter remains, like its Victorian predecessor, part of the repressive wing of the state. As such it contributes to the maintenance of social order by the use of lawfully devolved powers to suppress deviance. By contrast, the voluntary face of the mental health industry produces, with its willing participant patients, the prospect of life without distress. In the case of the psychotherapy client it creates reflective selves and normative clinical routines (Rose, 1990; de Swaan, 1990). In the case of some medicinal technologies this even extends to producing happiness, not just the removal of misery (Pilgrim and Dowrick, 2006).

Non-service factors relevant to the topic will now be considered.

What intergenerational and intragenerational effects are evident?

In chapter 7 the topic of age and mental health is explored. The argument is made clear that neglect and abuse in childhood have immediate implications for mental health inequalities and they have long-term consequences. Here another developmental effect to do with class of origin is noted. In Britain there have been two major longitudinal studies of relevance – the 1958 National Child Development Study (NCDS) and the 1970 British Birth Cohort Study (BCS). Sacker, School and Bartley (1999) summarize the implications for mental health and class position as follows:

▪ Both psychological problems and lower parental social class in adolescence increase the risk of mental health problems in adulthood (NCDS and BCS).

▪ The social position achieved in early adulthood is affected by both the father's class position and psychological problems in adolescence (NCDS and BCS).

▪ About 50 per cent of the relationship between social class and mental health status is accounted for by these pathways from parental social class position and adolescent mental health problems by the age of 23 (NCDS) and 26 (BCS). By the time the age of 33 is reached these two factors account for nearly 100 per cent of the relationship (NCDS).

▪ Mental health problems persist more from adolescence to adulthood in males than females (NCDS and BCS).

▪ Women show more intergenerational social mobility than men but intragenerational social mobility is the same for men and women (NCDS and BCS).

The greater persistence of problems in men from adolescence to adulthood is largely accounted for by behavioural or conduct disorders (substance misuse and chaotic and violent acting-out). Successful suicidal action is also greater in young males. Whether these differences are accounted for by testosterone or masculine identity (or both), other predictors from families of origin include low parental social class, urban living, domestic violence and physical chastisement (Regier *et al.*, 1988).

This link between male gender, low social class and acting out (violence to self and others) predicts higher rates of young men in *both* the penal system *and* secure parts of the mental health system. This general trend indicates a functional overlap between the criminal justice system and the mental health system. Both are aspects of the repressive wing of the state's apparatus of control. Both are used by government to control the disruptive aspects of the 'lumpen-proletariat' (the term used by Marx and Engels in their *German Ideology* of 1845) a concept implied more recently by that of the preferred notion of the 'underclass'. Both the old and new sociological terms have pejorative connotations. Marx at times called the lumpenproletariat social 'refuse' and 'flotsam' and saw them as parasitic and therefore dependent on the status quo, creating reactionary attitudes and habits to be distrusted. Chronic psychiatric patients would fall into this category.

Those with 'severe and enduring' mental health problems can be framed as one group within this broader underclass and so occupy an ambiguous socio-political space. They can be seen as part of a social threat and economic burden for the state and those in work. They can also be seen as part of a group which can now generate one of several forms of new social movement. The latter make demands for change in civil society to embrace diversity and equality (Habermas, 1981; Touraine, 1981). Accounts of the development of the mental health service-user movement can be found in Rogers and Pilgrim (2005) and Crossley (2006).

If social class predicts mental health problems and experiencing the latter maintains a lowly social position, is this just a matter of the uneven distribution of wealth in capitalist societies? This next section argues that money is important, but other forms of capital are also relevant.

What types of capital affect mental health?

Generally, the probability of a psychiatric diagnosis decreases with raised socio-economic position. The broad conclusion we can draw from this general trend is that being poor is bad for mental health, both as a causal factor and as a maintenance factor. However, the concept of poverty has become elaborated over time. In recent years sociological accounts of social exclusion or financial disadvantage have added to the traditional position about economic factors.

Apart from financial capital (income maintenance and savings), there is also an extensive discussion now of social capital and cultural capital. Financial capital is most readily described in *structural* terms as social class, defined by a combination of earnings and type of employment. Cultural and social capital are correlated with these variables but are better described in *functional or instrumental* terms – the ways and means people operate consciously or unconsciously to maintain or improve their social position, well-being and quality of life. Social class lends itself to objective indices but the other two also require descriptions, which capture subjective and intersubjective phenomena. The broader notion of 'socioeconomic status' rather than 'social class' implies all three forms of capital, but it emerged before the notions of cultural and social capital were properly developed.

All three types of capital can impinge on mental health status and vice versa. Poverty is a causal antecedent for some mental health problems and some mental health problems create economic disadvantage. But money is only part of the picture. With a poor family of origin (a risk factor in mental health problems) comes a sense of particular cultural space to do with locality, schooling and family expectations about social status and prospects. Personal identity and 'knowing one's place' are set early in childhood. This emphasis on developing a sense of one's place in life (Bourdieu, 1983) describes a person's 'cultural capital'. This is bound up with the later connectivity people develop with others as adults – their 'social capital'.

Cultural capital does not neatly prescribe the quality and amount of later social capital, but it does predict it. This is why intragenerational and intergenerational social mobility is possible but not probable for most. It was noted above that mental health problems in adolescence, along with low parental social class, are highly predictive of later mental health problems. This certainly suggests the importance of cultural capital as a source of psychosocial vulnerability for some people in society who are set on a trajectory of mental health problems. It combines with economic position to predict mental health status. By implication, those from better-off families who are also likely to have greater cultural capital are less prone to this trajectory.

Granovetter (1973) noted the bridge between cultural and social capital in the latter regard (who you know, not what you know). He described how social networks of better-off people involve multiple 'weak ties'. By contrast, poorer people have far less of these and tend to focus on the 'strong ties' of kith and kin. Bourdieu (1983) also elaborated the same points about networks of influence inhabited by richer people and which exclude poorer people. For Bourdieu we all inhabit different 'fields' (the economy, education, the family, the scientific world, etc.). Individuals tend to operate predominantly in one field but can move between them. Some of us have more opportunities than others in this regard. To be locked into one field denotes 'entrapment' – a concept that has been used at times to explain the emergence of both psychosis (Laing and Esterson, 1964) and depression (Brown, Harris and Hepworth, 1995).

Conceptually, Bourdieu contrasts 'field' with 'habitus'. The latter refers to our character, identity and habits arising from our past socialization and current immersion in social relationships. This distinction is similar to one of people and places, self and social context or even, more crudely, individual and society. These interactions are now explored by looking at the mental health implications of people and neighbourhoods.

What is the relationship between people and neighbourhoods?

Bourdieu's emphasis on 'field' and 'habitus' reminds us that subjectivity and intersubjectivity are bound up not only with who people are but where they are. At the same time this also points up the ecological fallacy; the socio-economic status of people is not *only* about where they live. A caution here then is that locality cannot be taken as a simple proxy from social class. For example, in poor, socially disorganized city localities some residents may be well off financially and relatively rich in both cultural and social capital. Nonetheless, some environmental neighbourhood effects may undermine the mental health of these better-off people, when they are compared with their peers in better-off localities. Thus, as we note now by summarizing some findings, the link between place and mental health is complicated. Mental health cannot be reduced to place but place does make a variable and sometimes substantial contribution. The following list captures this complexity.

- *Urban life generally is more stressful than rural life* (Li Wang, 2004; Paykel *et al.*, 2000). Urban life brings with it more social disorganization, environmental stressors (crime, vandalism, noise, litter and motor traffic) and concentrated areas of poverty. Health and well-being increase in country areas (but beware the ecological fallacy noted above – in rural localities, rich and poor live close to each other). In areas of concentrated poverty, which are socially disorganized, the impact at the individual level can be profound and negative. Not surprisingly, in these neighbourhoods there are raised levels of depression, anxiety and substance misuse (Aneschensel and Succoff, 1996). Apart from the direct exposure to the external 'ambient hazards' of stress described above, people in these local contexts are less likely to have regular supportive social networks, particularly if there is a high turnover of residence (Sampson, 1988).

- *Some diagnoses are more common in some localities.* This point was first noted in an early study from the ecological wing of the Chicago School of sociology around the time of the Second World War. Faris and Dunham found higher rates of diagnosed schizophrenia and substance misuse 'in the deteriorated regions and surrounding the centre of the city, no matter what race or nationality inhabited that region' (1939, 35). They went on to argue that the lack of social integration in these stressful, socially disorganized areas contributed to the 'confused, frustrated and chaotic' conduct associated with mental disorder. Later studies of the link between locality and mental health status confirmed these early indications (Smith, 1984).

- *There are specific and independent locality effects.* For example, some particular deteriorated localities contain higher rates of presentation of depressive symptomatology (Ross, 2000) *in all social groups*, including those with higher rates of forms of capital. Similarly, aggregate neighbourhood income predicts levels of diagnosis of schizophrenia and substance misuse (Goldsmith, Hoilzer and Manderscheid, 1998). People in poor areas defined at the individual level as being of the same socioeconomic status as those in richer areas are more likely to perpetrate and be victims of crime than their equivalents in richer areas (South and Crowder, 1997). This differential pattern about crime features is also evident when psychiatric patients with the same diagnosis are studied in rich and poor areas (Silver, 2000).

- *Some neighbourhoods provide more 'opportunity structures' than others.* These refer to the cultural and environmental possibilities for stress-free or health-giving public behaviour. For example, two neighbourhoods may be grossly equivalent in terms of income, but one may have safer streets and more spacious green park areas than the other. Generally though, more affluent neighbourhoods provide more opportunity structures than poorer ones (Ellaway and Macintyre, 1998). This emphasizes that social position can be defined as either an individual or a neighbourhood characteristic.

▪ *Opportunity structures interact with individual factors* (such as the three forms of capital and past mental health status) to create particular cultural landscapes. The latter will vary from place to place in terms of their life-enhancing or life-diminishing impact on local residents (Curtiss and Rees-Jones, 1998; Gesler, 1992). Thus framing this in terms discussed above from Bourdieu, the field of residency interacts with others that residents might occupy, as well as variations in the habitus of each individual in the neighbourhood.

▪ *Type of housing occupancy* predicts factors affecting mental health. Owner-occupiers show more self-esteem, mastery and life satisfaction than tenants in the same locality (MacIntyre, Maciver and Sooman, 1993).

The above, far from exhaustive, summary of locality and specific neighbourhood effects can be placed in a context of wider social policy. Given that poverty both increases the probability of mental health problems arising and exposes those already diagnosed to adverse stressors and social isolation, the extent to which poverty reduction measures from central and local government are present and effective is important. Moreover, in very deprived areas, manifesting concentrated poverty (and echoing the early Chicago School studies noted above), the incidence, not just the prevalence, of diagnosed schizophrenia is significantly higher (Boydell *et al.*, 2004; van Os *et al.*, 2002). This suggests that the social and environmental features of extreme poverty are not just relapse factors but are *causal* factors in psychosis. These neighbourhoods also have higher rates of dual diagnosis (psychosis and substance misuse). They increase the incidence of both psychotic symptoms and violence, with patients in these areas being at greater risk of being both victims and perpetrators in the latter regard (Todd *et al.*, 2004).

Finally in this section, it should be noted that mental health service users are more than less likely to return to conditions of poverty, although this effect is stronger in North America than in Europe because the former provides weaker economic support for those outside the labour market. As a consequence, Scull, commenting from the USA, argued that in the wake of desegregation, 'the alternative to the institution has been to be herded into newly emerging "deviant ghettoes", sewers of human misery ... conventionally defined as social pathology within which (largely hidden from outside inspection or even notice) society's refuse may be repressively tolerated' (Scull, 1977: 153).

This dramatic picture has not been as evident in Western Europe for users discharged from the old, large hospitals. However, there is a risk that without appropriate residency arrangements for newly emerging service users (i.e. young people who were never in the old hospitals), the picture could also gradually emerge on this side of the Atlantic. Mental health service users, like others outside the labour market, are found in areas of concentrated poverty, with a poor housing stock and high rates of rented property. These localities have effectively become 'service-dependent' ghettoes – a description that confirms Scull's picture but implicates a wider group of people (Dear and Wolch, 1987; Sayce, 2000; Wallace and Wallace, 1997). This suggests that apart from poverty reduction, housing policy is an important dimension of a genuine mental health policy.

How coherent is professional knowledge for our understanding of mental health in its social context?

The above exploration highlights a central difficulty with providing definitive answers to questions about the relationship between mental health and socio-economic disadvantage. Knowledge about this and any other aspect of mental health research is highly contested. This is not only a matter, as in many fields of enquiry, of differing interpretations of empirical findings. It is also about the concepts or constructs invoked or assumed *pre-empirically* and a failure to agree *non-empirically* about normative or moral assumptions. For example, pre-empirically, some researchers are confident about the conceptual validity of psychiatric diagnoses such as 'schizophrenia' or 'depression'. Others consider these concepts to have very weak conceptual validity and so they are deemed worthless for research purposes.

An example of non-empirical contestation relates to assumptions about the nature of madness. Is it a defect or a heightened state of consciousness? Should mad people be left alone or interfered with against their will? How these questions are answered matters. If madness is framed as an illness that implies warranted state and professional paternalism then psychiatric epidemiology would investigate the prevalence of 'schizophrenia' in order to plan appropriate levels of local mental health services. If not, then the latter would be irrelevant. For example, the radical edge of the users' movement has defended a counter-dependent position. They want fewer, not more, statutory services and they argue that madness has value – it is not pathology to be discounted, interfered with or controlled.

Any research agenda is shaped by a researcher's pre-empirical and non-empirical starting point. The latter determines which research questions they do or do not ask. Similarly, for students, reading and appraising literature will favour research, which makes sense in terms of their pre-empirical and non-empirical assumptions. When they read literature, which does not fit their assumptions, they will either discount it or be perplexed by it. These differing pre-empirical and non-empirical positions are very varied but largely coalesce around a few main epistemological positions. Elsewhere the range of perspectives on mental health inside and outside of sociology is examined (Rogers and Pilgrim, 2005). Some points will be made in concluding this chapter about some perspectives to examine in particular.

The first might be called 'medical naturalism' or 'psychiatric positivism'. It has been the mainstay position for the psychiatric profession and many in mental health nursing. Psychiatric diagnosis is deemed to be a valid description of what people who are mentally disordered say and do. But this is a circular logic. People are deemed to be schizophrenic because they hallucinate and have delusions. Their hallucinations and delusions are then accounted for by their schizophrenia. Undeterred by this tautology, the practical challenge ('the duty of care' supported by the medical 'right to treat') then is to provide treatments which reduce the symptoms of this putative mental disorder.

In accordance with medical naturalism, psychiatric epidemiology has become a matter of simply counting cases. These descriptive 'disease maps' even extend to behavioural events, such as suicide, which are dramatic but crude and even dubious proxies for mental health (Rezaeian *et al.*, 2004). By contrast, in its origins proper medical epidemiology traced the *causal* correlation between disease and its origins – the model worked at its best with infectious disease. Psychiatric epidemiology cannot do this because the cause of most mental disorders is contested or unknown. But it defines the need for services on the basis of this counting. This circularity seems to be driven by professional interest – investigations are pursued to demonstrate the need for professional services.

In earlier days (and this is the one genuine link with the social), when the psychiatric profession conceded the weak basis of its disease categories, *social correlates* were taken seriously (Pilgrim and Rogers, 2005). If germs could not be found to account for madness and misery, poverty, social isolation, trauma and loss might be more evident. At its best this model co-opted non-psychiatrists (Brown and Harris, 1978; Falloon and Fadden, 1993; Goldberg and Huxley, 1980) to form a multi-disciplinary project, 'social psychiatry'. However, the latter has more recently been replaced in psychiatric epidemiology by more narrow concerns about methodology and the sorts of justification for services noted above (Pilgrim and Rogers, 2005). Social psychiatry and a rump of sociologists within it remain the shaky bridge between psychiatry as a profession and sociology as an academic discipline, and leads to the next point.

Apart from George Brown, some other sociologists investigating mental health have left psychiatric knowledge untroubled. For example, Walter Gove and his colleagues did not join labelling theorists in questioning the benign value of professional action. Gove (1975, 1982) argued that psychiatric labelling, rather than contributing to personal invalidation and stigmatization, is a route into needed care for vulnerable people, whose deviance is driven from behind by their mental health problems not created by the actions of others, be they lay people or psychiatric professionals. However, the bulk of sociologists interested in mental health have considered that psychiatric theory and practice are not only about social control but also offer a body of knowledge, which does not properly capture the social. For this reason, many of the fellow-travellers of 'anti-psychiatry' in the 1960s were sociologists.

The problem with these criticisms from sociology about psychiatry is twofold. First, sociology itself is not of one voice when bidding to displace the shortcomings of medical knowledge. For example, a range of social theories from existentialism and symbolic interactionism to critical realism and social constructivism has informed sociological critiques of psychiatric positivism (Rogers and Pilgrim, 2005). Second, some of the most philosophically and socially trenchant critiques of psychiatry have come from psychiatrists themselves – initially the so-called 'anti-psychiatrists' and latterly the 'post-psychiatrists'. As a result, sociological criticisms of psychiatry can only legitimately focus on its bio-medical norms (the theory and practice of the bulk of its practitioners). Given the extensive, unrelenting and sophisticated criticisms emanating from a minor-ity of psychiatrists, stereotyping their profession from without is a risky business. For the same reason, the term 'anti-psychiatry' is misleading. The majority of critics under its label were psychiatrists and so the term is highly illogical, even though it remains common.

There are also overlaps and differences between all of these approaches to knowledge about mental health and social context. For example, despite their differences, versions of biological, psychological and sociological determin-ism share an assumption that causal relationships should define our field of inquiry. These versions of determinism to various degrees exclude the relevance of human agency in their accounts. By contrast, other forms of psychological and sociological account of mental health problems place agency at the centre.

Also, some approaches focus much more on consequences than causes. For example, labelling theory pays less attention than social causationism to antecedents of mental health problems and concentrates instead on the social negotiation of difference, exclusion and stigma. Similarly, some user groups like the Hearing Voices Network emphasize either the potential *intelligibil-ity* of madness or even celebrate its *superior* quality. For example, parts of the service-user movement like *Mad Pride* provide much material which depicts madness not as pathology or pitiable affliction but as a preferable escape from the conformity of a bourgeois moral order (Curtis *et al.*, 2004). Bentall (2004) cites Wittgenstein's query, 'madness need not be regarded as an illness. Why shouldn't it be seen as a sudden – more or less sudden – change of character?' This is another way of reframing mental illness.

These shifts of focus, about which form of knowledge to take seriously, are important. By moving towards intelligibility and celebration, do mental health problems effectively disappear? Once psychological differences are rendered understandable they are normalized and could be framed as not 'mental health problems' at all. The term 'mental health problems' has become a catch-all to replace the more dubious ones of 'mental illness' and 'mental disorder'. But these preferred semantic shifts still assume that overt psychological differ-ences, as judged by current cultural or societal norms, are problematic. And the term 'mental disorder' still covers two quite distinct groups of problematic conduct – one referring to problems to the self and another referring to prob-lems to others. In the former case self-labelling is all-important, whereas in the latter the attributions of others predominate (Thoits, 1985).

Strong versions of constructivism, from professional critics and radical users, challenge the assumption that forms of mental disorder have a self-evident sta-tus that can be validly described and measured. The problems of madness and misery, then, lie not inevitably in any inherent impairment of perception, emo-tion or conduct of identified patients. Instead they are located in the contexts they inhabit, particularly in intolerant norms and the fetish for rationality. Once this epistemological tack is taken then warranted paternalism to those with psychological afflictions melts away.

Conclusion

Taken as a whole, this is a confusing field for students of the topic. Which body of knowledge should be trusted? Should it be that of psychiatric epidemiology, with its confidence-inspiring 'facts' about correlations that seem to demonstrate links between social conditions and psychiatric diagnoses? Should it be that of 'anti-psychiatry' and the critical users who return, again and again, to psychiatry being part of the problem about, not the solution to, mental health and inequality? Should it be from sociologists and internal dissenters (the post-psychiatrists) who have abandoned epidemiology in favour of social constructivism (Bracken and Thomas, 2006)?

Each reader can situate him or herself within one of these groups, which approaches the topic from a different perspective to the others. They may even feel torn between them. What is not on offer at present is a simple body of knowledge that provides a coherent account under this chapter's heading to reassure and enlighten the student new to the topic. What is offered instead are some ways of thinking about it.

EDITORS' QUESTIONS

Issues of difference

- In what way can gender be an influence in economic status?
- What are the effects of unemployment on different age groups?
- Does culture define socioeconomic status?

Relevance to practice

- In what ways do you consider poverty when working in a mental health service?
- You discover a family have insufficient food. How do you respond as a health professional within your role?
- How can the multi-disciplinary team ensure the rights of a person with psychosis are upheld?

Investigate

- What are the forms of poverty, and how do they impact on mental health?
- How is the socioeconomic status of each service user determined?
- How do mental health professionals address unemployment in your team?

Suggested further reading

Dohrenwend, B.P. (ed.) (1998) *Adversity, Stress and Psychopathology*. Oxford: Oxford University Press.

Rogers, A. and Pilgrim, D. (2003) *Mental Health and Inequality*. Basingstoke: Palgrave Macmillan.

References

Alexander, L.A. and Link, B.G. (2003) The impact of contact on stigmatising attitudes toward people with mental illness. *Journal of Mental Health*, **12**(3), 271–90.

Andrea, H., Bultmann, U., Beurskens, A.J.H.M., Swaen, G.M.H., van Schayck, C.P. and Kant, I.J. (2004) Anxiety and depression in the working population using the HAD scale. *Social Psychiatry and Psychiatric Epidemiology*, **39**(8), 637–46.

Aneschensel, C.S. and Succoff, S. (1996) The neighbourhood context of mental health. *Journal of Health and Social Behaviour*, **37**, 293–311.

Bentall, R.P. (2004) *Madness Explained: Psychosis and Human Nature*. Harmondsworth: Penguin.

Bindman, J., Tighe, J., Thornicroft, G., and Leese, M. (2002) Poverty, poor services and compulsory psychiatric admission in England. *Social Psychiatry and Psychiatric Epidemiology*, **37**(7), 341–5.

Bourdieu, F. (1983) The forms of capital. In J. Richardson (ed.) *The Handbook of Theory and Research for the Sociology of Education*. New York: Greenwood.

Boydell, J., van Os, J., McKenzie, K., and Murray, R.M. (2004) The association of inequality with the incidence of schizophrenia: an ecological study. *Social Psychiatry and Psychiatric Epidemiology*, **39**(8), 597–9.

Bracken, P. and Thomas, P. (2006) *Postpsychiatry: Mental Health in a Postmodern World*. Oxford: Oxford University Press.

Brown, G. and Harris, T. (1978) *The Social Origins of Depression*. London: Tavistock.

Brown, G.W., Harris, T.O., and Hepworth, C. (1995) Loss, humiliation and entrapment among women developing depression: a patient and non-patient comparison. *Psychological Medicine*, **25**, 7–21.

Crossley, N. (2006) *Contesting Psychiatry*. London: Routledge.

Curtis, S. and Rees-Jones, I. (1998) Is there a place for geography in the analysis of health inequality? *Sociology of Health and Illness*, **20**(5), 546–73.

Curtis, T., Dellar, R., Leslie, E., and Watson, B. (2004) *Mad Pride: A Celebration of Mad Culture*. London: Spare Change Press.

Dear, M. and Wolch, J. (1987) *Landscapes of Despair: From Institutionalisation to Homelessness*. Oxford: Polity Press.

Delespaul, P., de Vries, M., and van Os, J. (2002) Determinants of occurrence and recovery from hallucinations in daily life. *Social Psychiatry and Psychiatric Epidemiology*, **37**(3), 97–104.

de Swaan, A. (1990) *The Management of Normality*. London: Routledge.

Dooley, D., Prause, J., and Ham-Rowbottom, K.A. (2000) Underemployment and depression: longitudinal relationships. *Journal of Health and Social Behaviour*, **41**, 421–36.

Ellaway, A. and Macintyre, S. (1998) Does housing tenure predict health in the UK because it exposes people to different levels of housing related hazards in the home or its surroundings? *Health and Place*, **4**, 141–50.

Falloon, I. and Fadden, G. (1993) *Integrated Mental Health Care*. Cambridge: Cambridge University Press.

Faris, R.E. and Dunham, H.W. (1939) *Mental Disorders in Urban Areas: An Ecological Study of Schizophrenia and Other Psychoses*. Chicago: Chicago University Press.

Fryer, D. (1995) Labour market disadvantage, deprivation and mental health. *The Psychologist*, **8**(6), 265–72.

Fryers, T., Melzer, D., and Jenkins, R. (2000) *Mental Health Inequalities Report 1: A Systematic Literature Review*. Cambridge University: Department of Public Health and Primary Care.

Gesler, W.M. (1992) Therapeutic landscapes: medical issues in the light of the new cultural geography. *Social Science and Medicine*, **34**(7), 735–46.

Goldberg, D. and Huxley, P. (1980) *Mental Illness in the Community*. London: Tavistock.

Goldsmith, H.F., Holzer, C.E., and Manderscheid, R.W. (1998) Neighbourhood characteristics and mental illness. *Evaluation and Program Planning,* **21**, 211–25.

Gove, W.R. (1975) The labeling theory of mental illness: a reply to Scheff. *American Sociological Review,* **40**, 242–8.

Gove, W.R. (1982) The current status of the labeling theory of mental illness. In W.R. Gove (ed.) *Deviance and Mental Illness.* Beverley Hills: Sage.

Granovetter, M. (1973) The strength of weak ties. *American Journal of Sociology,* **78**, 1360–80.

Habermas, J. (1981) New social movements. *Telos,* **48**, 33–7.

Ingleby, D. (1981) Understanding mental illness. In D. Ingleby (ed.) *Critical Psychiatry: The Politics of Mental Health.* Harmondsworth: Penguin.

Jenkins, R., Lewis, G., Bebbington, P., Brugha, T., Farrell, M., Gill, B., and Meltzer, H. (2003) The National Psychiatric Morbidity surveys of Great Britain: initial findings from the household survey. *Psychological Medicine,* **27**, 775–89.

Kasl, S.V., Rodrigues, E., and Lasch, K.E. (1998) The impact of unemployment on health and well being. In B.P. Dohrenwend (ed.) *Adversity, Stress and Psychopathology.* Oxford: Oxford University Press.

Knapp, M. (2001) The costs of mental disorder. In G. Thornicroft and G. Szmuckler (eds) *Textbook of Community Psychiatry.* Oxford: Oxford University Press.

Laing, R.D. and Esterson, A. (1964) *Sanity, Madness and the Family.* Harmondsworth: Penguin.

Li Wang, J. (2004) Rural-urban differences in the prevalence of major depression and associated impairment. *Social Psychiatry and Psychiatric Epidemiology,* **39**(1), 19–25.

Ludermir, A.B. and Lewis, G. (2003) Informal work and common mental disorders. *Social Psychiatry and Psychiatric Epidemiology,* **38**(9), 485–9.

Macintyre, S., Maciver, S., and Sooman, A. (1993) Area, class and health; should we be focusing on places or people? *Journal of Social Policy,* **22**, 213–34.

Marwaha, S. and Johnson, S. (2004) Schizophrenia and employment. *Social Psychiatry and Psychiatric Epidemiology,* **39**(5), 337–49.

Miller, P. and Rose, N. (1988) The Tavistock programme: the government of subjectivity and social life. *Sociology,* **22**(2), 171–92.

Patel, V. (2001) Poverty, inequality and mental health in developing countries. In D. Leon and G. Walt (eds) *Poverty, Inequality and Health.* Oxford: Oxford University Press.

Paykel, E.S., Abbott, R., Jenkins, R., Brugha, T.S., and Meltzer, H. (2000) Urban–rural mental health differences in Great Britain: findings from the National Morbidity Survey. *Psychological Medicine,* **30**(2), 269–80.

Pearlin, L.I. and Scaff, M.M. (1996) Stress and the life course: a paradigmatic alliance. *The Gerontologist,* **36**, 239–47.

Pilgrim, D. and Dowrick, C. (2006) From and diagnostic-therapeutic to a social existential response to 'depression'. *Journal of Public Mental Health* (in press).

Pilgrim, D. and Rogers, A. (2005) The troubled relationship between sociology and psychiatry. *International Journal of Social Psychiatry,* **51**(3), 228–41.

Regier, D. *et al.* (1988) Prevalence of mental disorders in the United States. *Archives of General Psychiatry,* **45**, 977–85.

Rezaeian, M., Dunn, G., St. Leger, S., and Appleby, L. (2004) The production and interpretation of disease maps: a methodological case study. *Social Psychiatry and Psychiatric Epidemiology,* **39**(12), 947–54.

Rogers, A. (1993) Coercion and voluntary admissions: an examination of psychiatric patients' views. *Behavioral Sciences and the Law,* **11**, 259–67.

Rogers, A. and Pilgrim, D. (2003) *Mental Health and Inequality.* London: Palgrave.

Rogers, A. and Pilgrim, D. (2005) *A Sociology of Mental Health and Illness* (3rd edn). Maidenhead: Open University Press.

Rose, N. (1979) The psychological complex: mental measurement and social administration. *Ideology and Consciousness*, **4**, 5–68.

Rose, N. (1986) Psychiatry: the discipline of mental health. In P. Miller and N. Rose (eds) *The Power of Psychiatry*. Cambridge: Polity Press.

Rose, N. (1990) *Governing the Soul*. London: Routledge.

Ross, C.E. (2000) Neighbourhood disadvantage and adult depression. *Journal of Health and Social Behaviour*, **41**, 177–87.

Ruesch, P., Graf, J., Meyer, P.C., Rossler, W., and Hell, D. (2004) Occupation, social support and quality of life in persons with schizophrenic or affective disorders. *Social Psychiatry and Psychiatric Epidemiology*, **39**(9), 686–94.

Sacker, A., School, I., and Bartley, M. (1999) Childhood influences on socio-economic inequalities in adult mental health: path analysis as an aid to understanding? *Health Variations*, **4**, 8–10. Lancaster: ESRC.

Sampson, R.J. (1988) Local friendship ties and community attachment. *American Sociological Review*, **53**, 766–79.

Sayce, L. (2000) *From Psychiatric Patient to Citizen: Overcoming Discrimination and Exclusion*. Basingstoke: Macmillan.

Scull, A.T. (1977) *Decarceration*. Englewood Cliffs NJ: Prentice Hall.

Silver, E. (2000) Race neighbourhood, disadvantage and violence amongst persons with mental disorders: the importance of contextual measurement. *Law and Human Behaviour*, **23**(2), 237–47.

Smith, D.M. (1984) Geographical approaches to mental health. In H.L. Freeman (ed.) *Mental Health and the Environment*. London: Churchill Livingstone.

South, S.J. and Crowder, K.D. (1997) Escaping distressed neighbourhoods: individual, community and metropolitan influences. *American Journal of Sociology*, **102**, 1040–84.

Szmuckler, G. and Appelbaum, P. (2001) Treatment pressures, coercion and compulsion. In G. Thornicroft and G. Szmuckler (eds) *Textbook of Community Psychiatry*. Oxford: Oxford University Press.

Thoits, P. (1985) Self labeling processes in mental illness. *American Journal of Sociology*, **91**, 221–49.

Tien, A.Y. (1991) Distribution of hallucinations in the population. *Social Psychiatry and Psychiatric Epidemiology*, **26**, 287–92.

Todd, J., Green, G., Harrison, M., Ikuesan, B.A., Self, C., Pevalin, D.J., and Baldacchino, A. (2004) Social exclusion in clients with comorbid mental health and substance misuse problems. *Social Psychiatry and Psychiatric Epidemiology*, **39**(7), 581–7.

Touraine, A. (1981) *The Voice and the Eye*. New York: Cambridge University Press.

Tudor-Hart, J. (1971) The inverse care law. *The Lancet*, **1**: 405–12.

van Os, J., Hanssen, M., Bijl, R.V., and Ravelli, A. (2000) Strauss (2000) revisited: a psychosis continuum in the normal population. *Schizophrenia Research*, **45**, 11–20.

van Os, J., Hansenn, M., de Graaf, R., and Vollebergh, W. (2002) Does the urban environment independently increase the risk for both positive and negative features of psychosis? *Social Psychiatry and Psychiatric Epidemiology*, **37**(10), 460–4.

Wallace, R. and Wallace, D. (1997) Socio-economic determinants of health: community marginalisation and the diffusion of disease and disorder in the United States. *British Medical Journal*, **314**, 1341.

Warner, R. (1985) *Recovery from Schizophrenia: Psychiatry and Political Economy*. London: Routledge.

Wilhelm, K., Kovess, V., Ross-Seidel, C., and Finch, A. (2004) Work and mental health. *Social Psychiatry and Psychiatric Epidemiology*, **39**(11), 866–73.

Institutional Racism and Cultural Diversity

Suman Fernando

BRIEF CHAPTER OUTLINE

Within this chapter psychiatry will be examined from a perspective of racism and cultural diversity. Brief terms of reference are offered, together with observations of mental health across cultures. The chapter then explores racism in the context of psychiatry being applied through imperial domination and suppression of non-western approaches. Service provision in the UK is reviewed for the concept of institutional racism and the rise of racial inequality, concluding by detailing ways in which psychiatry may overcome the issues discussed.

Introduction

The delivery of mental health services involves the participation of professionals from a variety of backgrounds and disciplines – psychiatry, social work, occupational therapy, clinical psychology and so on. But the main body of knowledge that informs all these disciplines and provides the backbone to the training of mental health professionals stems from psychiatry and clinical psychology. This chapter will focus on examining psychiatry in particular from a point of view of cultural diversity of the human race and racism linked to skin colour.

After a brief discussion on the terms culture, 'race' and ethnicity and the meanings of mental health and mental disorder from a transcultural perspective, the permeation of racism in psychiatry and western psychology will be illustrated by pointing to some theories that are recognisably racist, highlighting observations, often presented and accepted as 'facts', made over the years that show up underlying racist attitudes.

The second section of this chapter will argue that psychiatry has been applied across the globe on the back of scientific medicine and imperial domination. Consequently it has suppressed non-western approaches to mental health and to ways of dealing with problems that are termed (in western discourse) 'mental health problems' or 'mental illness'. In its application in contexts where the cultural influences are predominantly Asian or African, psychiatry imposes ways of thinking that are alien to the cultural norms of society, thus creating a culture clash between the services (based on psychiatry) and their users.

The third section will discuss briefly the concept of institutional racism, then review the problems that minority ethnic communities encounter when they come into contact with mental health services, problems usually referred to in the UK as 'ethnic issues'. The culture clash (already referred to) will be described. This is when Eurocentric psychiatry impacts on people from non-western backgrounds. Serious problems arise, identified as 'racial inequalities' in the case of service provision and 'cultural issues' in the case of theoretical formulations. It will be proposed that these problems and issues result from a combination of cultural insensitivity in professional practice, as well as institutional racism within psychiatry and psychology.

Finally, the chapter concludes by discussing ways in which psychiatry may overcome the impediments that arise from its ethnocentricity and the institutional racism embedded in it. It will argue that, if psychiatry is to have a beneficial role in a multicultural world composed of pluralistic societies (where imperialism and the domination of one cultural group over others is a fact of life), then it must be very different to that currently in vogue. Discussion will detail the road along which psychiatry needs to travel in arriving at something that eventually looks like and, more importantly, feels like a 'multicultural psychiatry'.

Categorization and terms of reference

The categorization of people on the basis of cultural background, (perceived) 'race' or (self-ascribed) ethnicity are interrelated in complex ways, depending on historical, political and social factors. In short, race is primarily physical, culture is sociological and ethnicity is psychological (Fernando, 2002). But the terms have become corrupted and misused over the years for a variety of reasons. A chapter such as this has to begin by clarifying how they are used – or should be – in a modern setting, for two reasons: By using the terms loosely or even interchangeably (as sometimes happens in many areas of thought, from politics to scientific research) what sometimes happens is that arguments become confused. But even more importantly, loose use of these terms may lead to the expression of prejudiced ideologies in covert form. An obvious example was in 1979 when the (then) leader of the British Opposition in the House of Commons, Margaret Thatcher, warned the electorate of being 'swamped' by alien cultures (quoted by Fitzpatrick, 1990: 249), when she clearly meant 'races' and not 'cultures'.

Mental health is a nebulous concept at the best of times. How this concept is best interpreted in the provision of mental health services in a multi-ethnic context is complicated. Clearly there is a need to look carefully at differences in the way mental health is seen in the diverse (cultural) traditions that comprise the particular society – broadly speaking, British society. But it is important to recognize similarities (between cultural traditions) as much as differences. Then, there should be awareness that cultures are not static; so the norms of 'tradition' may not necessarily apply to the here and now. Finally, it is important to be aware of the dangers of stereotyping people seen as 'belonging' to one or other ethnic group and of assumptions arising from popular perceptions about cultural background.

Culture, 'race' and ethnicity

The concept of 'race', meaning a biologically determined entity recognizable by one or two items of external appearance, usually skin colour, type of hair or shape of eyes (or a combination of these), has a long history in western Europe (see Dobzhansky, 1971; Molnar, 1983). Although dismissed in scientific biological circles as a basis for dividing up human beings into categories (Jones, 1981), the tendency to think of people in terms of their 'race' – 'race thinking' (Barzun, 1965) – persists for a variety of reasons – social, historical and psychological (Omi and Winant, 1994): 'The concept of race continues to play a fundamental role in structuring and representing the social world' (1994: 55).

Traditionally (for example in anthropological literature) 'culture' used to refer to non-material aspects of everything that a person holds in common with other individuals forming a social group (such as child-rearing habits, family systems, and ethical values or attitudes common to a group) described by Leighton and Hughes as 'shared patterns of belief, feeling and adaptation which people carry in their minds' (1961: 447) and which, in general, pass on from generation to generation. There was argument as to whether culture was 'something out there', a social concept, or something 'inside' a person (see D'Andrade, 1984). Today, culture is explored on a 'postmodern' terrain. It is no longer seen as something static inside or outside a person, but as something variable and relative, depending on historical and political viewpoints in a context of power relationships. *The Location of Culture* (Bhabha, 1994) emphasizes the hybridity of the concept in today's world. *Culture and Imperialism* (Said, 1994) unravels the intimate connections between the understandings of culture presented in Anglo-American literature and European domination – nowadays called 'globalization'. In general, culture is seen today as something that cannot be clearly defined, as something living, dynamic and changing – a flexible system of values and worldviews that people live by, a system by which they define identities and negotiate their lives (Fernando, 2002).

Strictly speaking, this postmodern concept of culture cannot be captured fully in terms of polarities such as East and West, traditional and modern. However, for practical purposes one has to resort to broad categories such as these in the interests of brevity for discussion and exploration. So, in practice, there is a tendency to regard a variety of items as indicative of a person's culture – sort of markers of culture, although these too are variable. They include main language or mother tongue; religious affiliation (or nominal religion); background in terms of heritage, values, loyalties, certain practices (say about food), dress codes and kinship ties; 'cultural' habits such as marriage preferences, world views and so on.

The term ethnicity alludes to self-perception of people in terms of 'belonging'. According to sociologist Stuart Hall, ethnicity 'acknowledges the place of history, language and culture in the construction of subjectivity and identity, as well as the fact that all discourse is placed positioned, situated, and all knowledge is contextual (1992: 257). However the bonds that bind people of an ethnic group together are not clearly definable in terms of physical appearance (race) or social similarity (culture) alone – although both may be involved. In practice, the sense of belonging – basically a psychological matter – may be promoted, or even initiated; by the way society at large perceives people. So, cultural similarity, real or imagined, may engender or even determine ethnicity. A sense (of belonging) may well arise for different reasons – for example, because the society in which they live treats them as a special group or as being (racially) 'different'.

In categorizing or describing people in terms of their culture, 'race' or ethnicity care must be taken as to what exactly is being talked about. Since the definition of culture is so variable and the subject of controversy, 'race' (based on observation) and ethnicity (based on self-designation) are used to define boundaries on the assumption – possibly an erroneous one – that culture is associated with one or the other. It is race that was used to enforce oppression through apartheid in South Africa with 'culture' being used as a justification. It is ethnicity that is used in the course of ethnic monitoring in order to locate (racial) discrimination in British employment practices. Yet there are real connections between culture, race and ethnicity. For example, the experience, post-slavery, of black people in the United States shaped a black consciousness – a sense of belonging to a group – as well as a recognizable black culture (Richardson and Lambert, 1985). In post-empire Britain, black people, sometimes finding themselves trapped into exclusion from British society, provided the base for a cultural revival of a 'West Indian consciousness' extending into a more generalized 'black consciousness' (Hall, 1978) or an 'Asianness'.

In a multiracial and multicultural society that is Britain today, ethnicity, identified by a sense of belonging, appears to be a useful concept for considering both social and mental health issues. Thus sociologists refer to 'new ethnicities' derived from African, Caribbean and Asian cultures in a context of complex social and cultural changes that have emerged in Britain's black and Asian communities during the past twenty years (Cohen, 1999). Differential experience of mental health services are analysed as 'ethnic differences' (see later). However, there needs to be an awareness that ethnicity emerges through various pressures – social, political, economic – and also cultural ties and perceptions of racial identity, the strength of which may be influenced by these same pressures. Ways in which ethnicity develops in twenty-first-century

British society depends on the significance of racism. If racism diminishes, the interplay of cultural diversity is likely to achieve increasing importance in determining ethnicity. But while racism continues racial difference will play an important part in determining ethnicity.

Mental health and disorder across cultures

The anthropological literature on transcultural psychiatry presents two basic approaches to the relationship between culture and health/illness – cultural relativity and cultural invariance (or universality). The former states that an understanding of health and illness is relative to each culture, with each culture having its own health and its own illness. The latter states that concepts of health and illness are universal, although culture determines the way illness is presented and problems of language, etc., lead to misunderstandings. The conflict between the cultural universalism (invariance) and cultural relativism continues in current thinking, usually in the form of an impasse. In the author's view, neither approach is acceptable today. First, biological, social and psychological influences determine the nature of what emerges as 'illness' in a particular cultural setting. Social construction of illness within a cultural context is important but not the only consideration. Second, as argued earlier, cultures are not distinct and unchanging. There is constant interchange between cultures, although powerful forces influence the nature of these changes – economic pressures, racism and even military might, to name just a few, all intertwined together.

The boundary between mental health and mental disorder (or illness) is concerned with the question of normality – a subject of much controversy (Offer and Sabshin, 1966), even within the limited domain of western culture. Once questions of cultural diversity are introduced, the issues are magnified several fold. There is a need to (a) recognize that cultures develop their own norms for health, for ideal states of mind and for what is considered correct functioning of individuals in society; and (b) take on board the fact that the study of these 'cultural' norms may be distorted by prejudiced – often racist – perceptions of the cultures and people associated with those cultures. For example, varieties of inner experience acceptable as desirable states of consciousness within the cultures of Asia, Africa and pre-Columbian America may be perceived in the West as 'abnormal' experiences, even as 'illness'. Professionals from a western cultural tradition that places a special value on early separation of children from their parents may perceive close family ties between grown-up children and their parents in non-western families as (pathological and undesirable) enmeshment.

Not only is the concept of illness different across cultures but also the ways in which illnesses are perceived – the explanatory models for illness (Kleinman, 1980). In western culture, insanity is 'set apart' as a special type of illness – something that does not apply in the same way in many other cultures. In any case, understandings of insanity and 'mind' are often very different across cultures. Boundaries between health and disease and mind and body are drawn in different ways in different cultural traditions (see Fernando, 2002). As a result, the major causes of 'mental illness' (in western terms) may appear to be somato-psychic when classical Ayurvedic theories of Indian medicine are studied using western concepts (Obeyesekere, 1977); and some forms of human distress that are conceptualized in the West as 'illness' may be seen in religious or philosophical terms in the Indian tradition. In Tibetan thinking, based on Buddhist culture, the most crucial psychological factor involved with insanity is the same as that essential for pursuing enlightenment, namely, the recognition of impermanence (Clifford, 1984). Although the western model of illness has developed in a Christian culture, it has no place for Christian concepts such as 'salvation or 'damnation', because, in the West, religion and illness are now in separate cultural compartments. This secular approach to illness is not seen in other cultural traditions. The overall worldview within a culture, appertaining to health, religion, psychology and spiritual concerns, determines the meaning within that culture of 'madness', mental illness and mental health.

Racism in psychiatry

In his analysis of the connection between racism and colonialism, psychiatrist Frantz Fanon has shown how 'vulgar racism in its biological form' (1967: 35), corresponding to a period of crude exploitation, changed into 'cultural racism' – 'a more sophisticated form [of racism] in which the object is no longer the physiology of the individual but the cultural style of a people' (McCulloch, 1983:120). This form of racism, deeply embedded in European culture, is represented in western social and political systems as institutional racism of modern times (see below). Its manifestation in the psychiatric system is complex. A few examples are identified to illustrate how racism has permeated psychiatry over the years.

In the nineteenth century, psychiatrists in the United States argued for the retention of slavery, quoting statistics allegedly showing that mental illness was more often reported among freed slaves compared to those who were still in slavery (Thomas and Sillen, 1972). And it was at that time that Cartwright (1851) postulated that black slaves who persistently ran away suffered from a disease of the mind called *drapetomania,* named after Greek words meaning 'runaway slave' and 'mad or crazy'. When John Langdon Down (1866) surveyed so-called 'idiots' and 'imbeciles' resident in institutions around London, he identified them as 'racial throwbacks' to Ethiopian, Malay and Mongolian racial types – mostly, he said, they were 'Mongols'. He was in fact reflecting an explanation for pathology that was common at the time – the ideology of 'degeneration' (Morel, 1852). Historian Daniel Pick (1989: 37) believes that the concept of degeneration must primarily be understood within the language of nineteenth-century racist imperialism; the underlying thesis was that social conflict, aggression, insanity and criminality were all signs of individual pathology representing reversal (throwback) to a racially primitive stage of development, either mentally or physically, or both.

The idea that black people are underdeveloped white people underlies many theories and observations made by psychiatrists and psychologists throughout the twentieth century. When Kraepelin (1904) observed that guilt was not seen in Javanese people who became depressed, his conclusion was that the Javanese were 'a psychically underdeveloped population' akin to 'immature European youth' (Kraepelin, 1921: 171). Stanley Hall (1904), founder of the *American Journal of Psychology* and first president of the American Psychological Association (Thomas and Sillen, 1972: 7), described in a standard text on adolescence Asians, Chinese, Africans and Indigenous Americans as psychologically 'adolescent races' who 'live a life of feeling emotion and impulse' (1904: 80). Swiss psychologist Carl Jung observed that white Americans were culturally different to (white) Europeans because they were affected by 'racial infection' from living too close to black people. 'The inferior man exercises a tremendous pull upon civilized beings who are forced to live with him because he fascinates the inferior layers of our psyche' (Jung, 1930: 196).

The apparent rarity of depression among Africans and African Americans ('black people'), reported well into the 1950s (Prince, 1968), was attributed to their 'irresponsible' and 'unthinking' nature (Green, 1914) or their absence of 'a sense of responsibility for [their] past' (Carothers, 1953: 148). In other words, their underdevelopment. Leff (1973, 1981), after analysing observations across the world, concluded that people from Africa and Asia as well as black Americans (the politically 'Black') have a less developed ability to differentiate emotions when compared with Europeans and white Americans – a finding interpreted by him as representing the 'historical development of emotional differentiation', an 'evolutionary process' (1981: 65–6). Of course, these ideas are in line with recurring versions of the racist IQ movement (e.g. Herrnstein and Murray, 1994).

Twenty-first-century Britain, like many other western societies, is culturally diverse and institutional racism tends to be manifested in ideas and discourse about 'culture'. As Paul Gilroy points out, British racism now 'frequently operates without any overt reference to "race" itself or the biological notions of difference which still give the term its common-sense meaning' (1993: 23). 'Culture', as an immutable, fixed property of social groups, has become confounded with 'race', and racism is articulated in cultural terms.

The global imposition of psychiatry

A variety of cultural traditions are discernible across the world, some very different to others. Yet there has always been an intermingling of cultures and in today's world 'culture' cannot be considered as a static entity by any means. The overall thrust of cultural and social change globally since the early sixteenth century has been determined by power – mainly military power linked to a political will to dominate. Generally speaking, during the past five hundred years this has meant western domination, allied to skin-colour racism. As western influence spread, western ideas, technology and politics were imposed upon, or taken on by, Asian and African countries. western medical systems were favoured over all other systems and then achieved dominance by bringing about massive improvements in health wherever they were applied. And psychiatry, seen as a part of western medicine, has followed suit in being applied as a 'medical' system. In other words, the fact that psychiatry itself has never been shown to be applicable cross-culturally in any meaningful way or to be free of either racial or cultural bias has become obscured by its overt attachment to medicine – the prestige of the latter rubbing off on to psychiatry.

Today, psychiatry and the medical-type model of 'mental illness' take precedence over other (culturally speaking) more appropriate ways of conceptualizing human problems. What has happened is that, like all things western, psychiatry too is seen as 'modern', 'scientific' and superior to non-western indigenous ways of conceptualizing and dealing with (what in western terms are called) mental health problems. More recently, another force that has pushed psychiatry on to non-western countries is the promotion of drugs manufactured in the West and the consequent economic advantages to multinational companies with shareholders in the West controlling much of the economies of Asia and Africa.

The asylum movement in the West was a result of social and political conditions peculiar to western development, but it stayed to fashion much of the thinking in the West about 'insanity'. The asylum approach was imposed in countries which were colonised and/or dominated by European nations such as Britain, France and the Netherlands, so that mental hospitals in Asia and Africa are little different from those in Europe. Thus the institutional 'medical-illness' approach to the control of 'mad' people taken over from the West continues virtually unaltered with no regard to the social consequences of doing so, although such an approach was, and is, alien to the traditions of most non-western cultures.

One would imagine that changes in ways of working within mental health systems in Asia and Africa should come about today through sensitivity to indigenous cultures. Also, there is widespread challenge to the scientific status of psychiatry, summarized recently by Mezzina (2005) in the book *Mental Health at the Crossroads* (Ramon and Williams, 2005). But this is not occurring to any great extent, for two main reasons. First, there are political pressures to westernize services linked to overt western influence through 'aid'. Second, the indirect imposition of psychiatry takes place through training, advice by western 'experts' and the promotion by western pharmaceutical companies of drug therapy that is dependent on a medical frame of reference. The result of all this is that mental health services in the ex-colonial countries of Asia and Africa continue to be staffed by professionals trained in western methods of psychiatry alone, looking to drug therapies as a 'scientific' approach to the alleviation of mental distress and increasingly social problems medicalized as 'illness'. Bolstering the reinforcement of western psychiatry in Asia and Africa are the research projects backed by resources (derived in the West) which promote psychiatry and the illness approach to mental health. Thus, by using models and systems devised in politically powerful western 'centres of excellence' and backed by the prestige and finance of powerful organizations, indigenous systems of psychology, philosophy and medical care are stifled in the name of modernization and development. And, just as in the empires of the nineteenth and early twentieth centuries, ethnically indigenous professionals run the systems that oppress their own people.

An example of the problems presented by the global imposition of psychiatry may be seen in the case of 'depression'. The illness called depression arose from that of 'melancholia,' which goes back in western culture to the time of Hippocrates (Jones, 1823). But the validity of the current understanding of depression as an illness in other cultures is very dubious. Reviews of cross-cultural research based on the imposition of a western model of depression (as an illness), such as that by Singer (1975), produce the inevitable conclusion that a 'core illness' of depression is universally recognizable. But it is not just this 'core' illness that is diagnosed as depression. Marsella (1978) suggests that since the 'clinical picture' of the condition varies so much cross-culturally, depression as understood in psychiatric circles should be regarded as a disorder of the western world alone. Taking the alleged reports that 'depression' in non-European cultures is characterized by somatic symptoms rather than 'psychic' ones, he argues that, if depression is essentially an experience, a psychologically experienced 'depression' is different from one associated with somatic experience.

While acknowledging that 'a painful series of affects pertaining to sorrow' may be universally identifiable, the anthropologist Gananath Obeyesekere (1985) believes that it is illogical to assume that a constellation of symptoms reflecting this situation is a universal illness just because it has been designated as such in western culture. He argues that if a constellation identified in Asian cultures, such as weight loss, sexual fantasies, night emissions and urine discoloration (designated in parts of Asia as the illness of 'semen loss'), is identifiable in other cultures, a contention that it is therefore a universal illness would be 'laughed out of court'. He sees the fault in the methods of psychiatric epidemiology where 'symptoms are treated in isolation from their cultural context. 'While it is true that the disarticulation of symptoms from context will facilitate measurement, it is also likely that the entities being measured are empty of meaning' (1985: 137). The wider fault is in the context in which research is generally carried out with western backing. Although the fact that different cultures devise illnesses differently is often accepted, illness models derived from experience in western countries and western cultural contexts are paramount and supersede others whenever possible. For example, a review of depression by Bebbington (1978) refers to non-western presentations of the 'illness' as 'anomalies'. The underlying ethos may be conceptualized as cultural arrogance, white superiority or just racism.

The deleterious effects of imposing western 'mental illness' models across the globe is seen more recently in the medicalization of trauma during disasters, particularly common in the non-western world. Personal distress, normally dealt with in religious modes or as problems within family and social systems, is being forced into illness modes to be treated by manufactured drugs or psychotherapies developed in an alien culture. This was a particular problem after the tsunami that devastated parts of Sri Lanka and Indonesia in December 2004. Although the help provided by western agencies was invaluable, some problems were created as a result of psychologists and psychiatrists descending on vulnerable populations of bereaved people offering 'trauma counselling' based on techniques devised in a western cultural context and delivered without much sensitivity to local cultural traditions and norms (see Fernando, 2003). In some instances their interventions appeared to retraumatize people and generally cause more harm than good. Indeed the use of the western model of 'post-traumatic stress disorder' in non-western settings and for refugees from Asia and Africa who have sought asylum in the West has been strongly criticized (Summerfield, 2001).

What is being described is the imperialism of psychiatry – an imperialism that is less obvious than western military domination of Asia and Africa in the nineteenth and first half of the twentieth centuries and its economic counterpart of the second half of the twentieth and twenty-first centuries; however, it is no less powerful and destructive to the vast majority of people in the world. In the past, it has resulted in the imposition of the 'lunatic asylum' as a way of dealing with 'madness'. In the future, it will no doubt result in the imposition of other, equally alien, systems of 'care' derived in the West for 'psychiatric cases' – defined in western terms. That is, unless something is done about the relentless west-ernisation of the world (Harrison, 1979) currently taking place and carrying psychiatry with it.

Institutional racism in the West

The concept of institutional racism was first introduced in the 1960s in the context of the US civil rights movement by Stokely Carmichael and Charles Hamilton in separating overt 'racist' acts by individuals from a racism that was 'less overt, far more subtle, less identifiable in terms of specific individuals committing the [racist] acts'. This second type of racism, 'originating in the operation of established and respected forces in the society' (1967: 20), relies on a 'racist attitude that permeates society, on both the individual and institu-tional level, covertly and overtly' (1967: 20–1).

Racial prejudice is easy to recognize and generally something considered abhorrent in most civilized societies. But institutional racism by its very nature is often missed completely or excused as just 'normal' behaviour. Institutional racism is a useful concept to subsume expressions of racial discrimination and oppression in subtle ways that are not easily obvious or even appreciated by those who are involved. This is especially so in systems such as education and mental health, including the psychiatric system. The report of the inquiry into the investigation by the police into the murder of black teenager, Stephen Lawrence (Home Department, 1999), in South London in 1993 defined institutional racism as: 'the collective failure of an organisation to provide an appropriate and professional service to people because of their colour, culture or ethnic origin ... It can be seen or detected in processes, attitudes and behav-iour that amount to discrimination through unwitting prejudice, ignorance, thoughtlessness and racist stereotyping that disadvantages minority ethnic people' (1999: 28). Today institutional racism and racial prejudice at a personal level exist together, interacting with each other and affecting society in many different ways, changing their guise according to context. Racism is best seen as an influence that permeates a system, hitching on to anything suitable for its purposes, any ideology, any discrimination, any facet of social functioning, any system of care, any educational enterprise, any construction of knowledge. So racism, or perhaps racisms, takes diverse forms. The 'everyday racism' described by Essed (1990) merges into racial harassment and racial attacks. Although it may be the case that overt racial discrimination at a personal level (street racism) has declined over the past ten years in Britain, it is still experienced in varying degrees by many black people in their everyday interactions with others. But it is racism implemented through institutional processes, institutional racism, that is proving most difficult to address. These issues are discussed more fully elsewhere (Fernando, 2003).

Black people in the mental health system

The overrepresentation of black people among those compulsorily detained in psychiatric institutes and among people diagnosed as, 'schizophrenic' by psychiatrists has been known for over twenty years (see Fernando, 1988, 2003). Also, when compared to people from white ethnic groups, people from black and minority ethnic (BME) communities are less likely to be referred for 'talking therapies' and usually feel more dissatisfied with mental health services (see Fernando, 2003). A recent report on a study of the perceptions of black people who use mental health services found that 'circles of fear' leading to breakdown in trust, cultural insensitivity of professionals (both black and white professionals) and inappropriateness of the psychiatric system of diagnosis and treatment all play a part (Keating *et al.*, 2002). Ethnic differences seen in institutional settings within the National Health Service are much less obvious in community settings (Sproston and Nazroo, 2002). This supports a view that much of the problem arises from institutional factors. Since institutional practices in the mental health system arise primarily from psychiatry and western psychology, the problems are likely to be located largely, though not entirely, within these disciplines. So there is a need to examine them in terms of their ideologies, assumptions and ways of working.

Racial stereotyping

Through the use of psychiatric diagnosis, the basic approach in western psychiatry is to create categories – or 'typifications' (Schwartz and Wiggins, 1987), generalizations about individuals perceived as similar in some way. Also, these are constructed on the basis of theories and observations of the people interpreted (from a particular cultural perspective), ignoring the prejudices and assumptions about people inherent in such assumptions. It is easy for such categories to be or become stereotypes. Stereotypes, like categories, are generalizations, but they tend to supersede or deny individuality in a more definitive manner. Allport (1954) believed the former to be more fixed (than categories) and imbued with a judgemental quality. Also, a stereotype tends to be sustained even in the face of evidence that should really result in its abandonment. In that sense, they are akin to beliefs held against all evidence to the contrary – the definition of 'delusions', in psychiatric terminology.

Stereotypes often acquire a power of their own. Allport sees them as being 'socially supported, continually revived and hammered in, media of mass communication' (1954: 195). Thus, stereotypes can become very powerful determinants of the way social systems impinge on ordinary people and may play an important role in maintaining social inequalities and inequalities between people perceived as belonging to different 'race', resulting then in 'racial inequalities'. This is racist stereotyping. It may be supposed that the power of racist stereotyping will diminish as overt racism is suppressed or loses its importance. This is not usually the case. Racist stereotyping as a social force can exist even when overt racism is not evident. In fact it can become even more significant in the absence of overt racism. Pieterse (1992) points out that racist stereotyping increased after the abolition of slavery. And this is the case in psychiatry.

It was shown earlier that 'putting people away', designating them as 'alien' to normal humanity, is one of the primary functions of psychiatry as a system. Indeed, custodial care was the norm for a long time in the asylums. It was on the basis of the right to be custodians that psychiatrists, formerly called 'alienists', began to develop their systems of diagnosis. In modern psychiatry the 'putting-away' function is represented by the procedure of risk assessment. This, together with diagnosis, is a combination that is the bedrock of psychiatric power. In a context of racism, racist stereotyping is almost inevitable in the course of making mental health assessments (for diagnosis) and risk assessments, unless specific measures are taken to make sure they do not. Mental health professionals who are aware of this danger may take such an anti-racist approach in making mental health assessments and judgements of 'risk', but these are few and far between. The result is that institutional racism is at the very centre of the psychiatric process (diagnosis) and lies within the very substance of one of the main planks on which psychiatry rests for its power, making assessments of whether someone is 'at risk' or a danger to others.

Differentiating stereotypes from categories is an important aspect of the art of psychiatry and one that should be a part of psychiatric training. But of course this is not the case. Something that is coming into psychiatric training is 'cultural capability' training. Essentially this consists of enabling professionals to be 'culturally sensitive', a sensitivity that may involve appreciation of personal prejudice. But sensitivity itself, with knowledge of the racism that is integral to some of the fundamentals of the discipline, may do more harm than good. People trained in 'cultural sensitivity' may wrongly feel competent in dealing with race issues, erroneously conflating the concepts of 'race' and 'culture'. But more importantly, other people may wrongly make the assumption that they are competent in this way and so given authority.

Towards a multicultural psychiatry

Psychiatry has now been going in its present form for over one hundred years, if the Kraepelin era is taken as its start. Quite early on there were dissenting voices objecting to its basic premises from anthropologists (see Gaines, 1992) and later transcultural psychiatrists (see Kleinman, 1988). There have always been serious critiques of psychiatry for the past half-century, both within the discipline (see Ingleby, 2004), or on its fringes and outside it (see Ramon and Williams, 2005). More recently, a critique of psychiatry has emerged quoting racism within the discipline and society at large as an important issue (see Littlewood and Lipsedge, 1992; Fernando, 2003). All these critiques come together when considering how psychiatry should and must change if it is to survive as a discipline that is geared to serve the needs of people who are perceived as suffering mental health problems in the real world of today. A world composed of people who come from diverse cultural backgrounds and traditions, but who are becoming more and more involved with each other (in 'globalization').

This section refers briefly to three types of fundamental change that psychiatry has to undertake. All of these will carry immense complications and would attract resistance from various sources. Indeed it would require a revolution of sorts for such changes to take place. And revolution has its own problems, often betraying the very aims that its protagonists envisage. Gradual evolution, a journey as it were, is to be preferred. The first steps in such a journey may vary from place to place and person to person. In a recent book (Fernando, 2003), some of these first steps are outlined and the next three paragraphs outline the ultimate outcome.

Until now psychiatry has its roots in western European culture. It is necessary therefore for psychiatry to 're-root' itself in a plethora of world cultures or at least revise its fundamental ideologies by drawing from a plethora of world cultures. How is this to be achieved? The narrow western approach to mental illness and mental health must be re-examined. The psychologies that have dominated the world outside western Europe have thrived often as 'religion' (Buddhist psychology) or philosophy (e.g. Hindu philosophy) or spirituality (e.g. 'shamanism of pre-Columbian America). These must become mainstream within the discipline. Psychiatry needs to look to non-western systems of medicine, for example, Ayurveda (India), Chinese traditional medicine (TCM), and African systems (pejoratively and unjustly termed 'witchcraft' by western anthropologists) for inspiration in revising its theoretical base.

Since psychiatry comes from a western European social context, the racism that pervades psychiatry comes from that culture. Therefore the racism discussed in this chapter is much to do with colour racism. But the racisms that pervade non-western societies may not be identical with that in mainly white western societies. Clearly these other forms of racism that have generated conflict in many regions from Sri Lanka to Rwanda may need to be addressed when psychiatry is practised in the course of providing mental health services. And so a system to counteract racism that can be applied all over the world must be incorporated into a psychiatry that has worldwide applicability.

It would be evident from earlier sections of this chapter that the important issue regarding international imposition of psychiatry (through mental health systems) is one of power and imperialism that is implemented through psychiatry. The 'medical' status of psychiatry is the primary problem in this case. The remedy, then, is simple, although likely to have far-reaching consequences if acted upon. Psychiatry needs to be 'de-recognised' as a medical discipline. If it is reformed into a social enterprise, like, say, education or social welfare, then its application would naturally be variable depending on the social context in which it is practised. This means that mental health services are seen as social care services devoid of a 'medical' input except when there is specific (physical) illness involved. Such a transformation of psychiatry would inevitably have to apply worldwide, to the West as much as to the rest of the world.

So the message to end this chapter is that far-reaching and fundamental changes are required for psychiatry to become a humane, socially acceptable and just system that can inform and sustain services that may help people with mental health problems. The sooner the journey is started towards that goal the better.

EDITORS' QUESTIONS

Issues of difference

- In what way are black female service users discriminated against?
- What are the generational experiences within the UK black community?
- How could we embrace cultural diversity within mental health care?

Relevance to practice

- How do mental health professionals communicate concern for racism?
- How do we ensure cultural diversity in the mental health workforce?
- Should racial match be a concern amongst the professional disciplines?

Investigate

- What are the forms of discrimination?
- How is culture incorporated into the assessment within your service or practice?
- What are the key elements for identifying and preventing institutional racism within mental health services?

Suggested further reading

Fernando, S. (2003) *Cultural Diversity, Mental Health and Psychiatry: The Struggle against Racism*. Hove and New York: Brunner-Routledge.
Ingleby, D. (2004) *Critical Psychiatry. The Politics of Mental Health* (2nd rev. edn). London: Free Association Books.

References

Allport, G. (1954) *The Nature of Prejudice*. New York: Doubleday.
Barzun, J. (1965) *Race: A Study of Superstition*. New York: Harper & Row, cited in C. Husband (ed.) *Race in Britain: Continuity and Change*. London: Hutchinson, 1982, pp. 11–23.
Bebbington, P.E. (1978) The epidemiology of depressive disorder. *Culture, Medicine and Psychiatry*, **2**, 297–341.

Bhabha, H. (1994) *The Location of Culture*. London: Routledge.

Carmichael, S. and Hamilton, C.V. (1967) *Black Power: The Politics of Liberation in America*. New York: Random House.

Carothers, J.C. (1953) *The African Mind in Health and Disease: A Study in Ethnopsychiatry*. WHO Monograph Series No. 17. Geneva: World Health Organization.

Cartwright, S.A. (1851) Report on the diseases and physical peculiarities of the negro race. *New Orleans Medical and Surgical Journal*, **May**, 691–715.

Clifford, T. (1984) *Tibetan Buddhist Medicine and Psychiatry: The Diamond Healing*. York Beach, ME: Samuel Weiser.

Cohen, P. (1999) *New Ethnicities, Old Racisms?* London: Zed Books.

D'Andrade, R.G. (1984) Cultural meaning systems. In R.A. Shweder and R.A. LeVine (eds) *Cultural Theory: Essays on Mind, Self and Emotion*. Cambridge: Cambridge University Press, pp. 88–119.

Dobzhansky, T. (1971) Race equality. In R.H. Osborne (ed.) *The Biological and Social Meaning of Race*. San Francisco: Freeman, pp. 13–24.

Down, J.L.M. (1866) Observations on an ethnic classification of idiots: lectures and reports from the London Hospital for 1866. Reprinted In C. Thompson (ed.) *The Origins of Modern Psychiatry*. Chichester: Wiley, 1987, pp. 15–18.

Essed, P. (1990) *Everyday Racism* (2nd edn). Trans. C. Jaffé. Alameda, CA: Hunter House. Originally published in Dutch as *Alledaags Racisme*, Baarn, Netherlands: Ambo b.v.

Fanon, F. (1967) Racism and culture. Text of Franz Fanon's speech before the first congress of Negro writers and artists, Paris, September 1965, published in the special issue of *Présence Africaine*, June–November 1956. In F. Maspéro (ed.) *Toward the African Revolution: Political Essays*. Trans. H. Chevalier. New York: Grove Press, pp. 31–44.

Fernando, S. (1988) *Race and Culture in Psychiatry*. London: Croom Helm. Reprinted London, Routledge, 1989.

Fernando, S. (2002) *Mental Health, Race and Culture* (2nd edn). Basingstoke: Palgrave Macmillan.

Fernando, S. (2003) *Cultural Diversity, Mental Health and Psychiatry: The Struggle against Racism*. Hove and New York: Brunner-Routledge.

Fitzpatrick, P. (1990) Racism and the innocence of law. In D.T. Goldberg (ed.) *Anatomy of Racism*. Minneapolis: University of Minnesota Press, pp. 247–62.

Gaines, A. (ed.) 1992 *Ethnopsychiatry: The Cultural Construction of Professional and Folk Psychiatries*. Albany: State University of New York Press.

Gilroy, P. (1993) *Small Acts: Thoughts on the Politics of Black Cultures*. London: Serpent's Tail.

Green, E.M. (1914) Psychoses among negroes – a comparative study. *Journal of Nervous and Mental Disorder*, **41**, 697–708.

Hall, S. (1978) Racism and reaction. In Commission for Racial Equality (ed.) *Five Views of Multi-Racial Britain*. London: CRE, pp. 23–35.

Hall, S. (1992) New ethnicities. In J. Donald and A. Ratansi (eds) *'Race', Culture and Difference*. London: Sage, pp. 252–9.

Harrison, P. (1979) *Inside the Third World: The Anatomy of Poverty*. Harmondsworth: Penguin.

Herrnstein, R.J. and Murray, C. (1994) *The Bell Curve: Intelligence and Class Structure in American Life*. New York: Free Press.

Home Department (1999) *The Stephen Lawrence Inquiry: Report of an Inquiry by Sir William Macpherson of Cluny*. CM4262-I. London: Stationery Office.

Ingleby, D. (2004) *Critical Psychiatry. The Politics of Mental Health* (2nd rev. edn). London: Free Association Books.

Jones, J.S. (1981) How different are human races? *Nature*, **293**, 188–90.

Jones, W.H.S. (1823) *Hippocrates with an English Translation*. London: Heinemann.

Jung, C.G. (1930) Your Negroid and Indian behaviour. *Forum*, **83**(4), 193–9.

Keating, F., Robertson, D., McCulloch, A., and Francis, E. (2002) *Breaking the Circles of Fear. A Review of the Relationship between Mental Health Services and African and Caribbean Communities.* London: Sainsbury Centre for Mental Health.

Kleinman, A. (1980) Major conceptual and research issues for cultural (anthropological) psychiatry. *Culture, Medicine and Psychiatry,* **4**, 3–13.

Kleinman, A. (1988) *Rethinking Psychiatry. From Cultural Category to Personal Experience.* New York: The Free Press.

Kraepelin, E. (1904) Vergleichende Psychiatrie. *Zentralblatt Nervenheilkunde und Psychiatrie,* **27**, 433–7, trans. H. Marshall. In: S. R. Hirsch and M. Shepherd (eds) *Themes and Variations in European Psychiatry.* Bristol: Wright, 1974, pp. 3–6.

Kraepelin, E. (1921) *Manic-depressive Insanity and Paranoia,* trans. and ed. R.M. Barclay and G. M. Robertson. Edinburgh: Livingstone.

Leff, J. (1973) Culture and the differentiation of emotional states. *British Journal of Psychiatry,* **123**, 299–306.

Leff, J. (1981) *Psychiatry around the Globe.* New York: Dekker.

Leighton, A.H. and Hughes, J.H. (1961) Cultures as causative of mental disorder. *Millbank Memorial Fund Quarterly,* **39**(3), 446–70.

Littlewood, R. and Lipsedge, M. (1992) *Aliens and Alienists: Ethnic Minorities and Psychiatry* (2nd edn). London: Unwin Hyman.

Marsella, A.J. (1978) Thought on cross-cultural studies on the epidemiology of depression. *Culture, Medicine and Psychiatry,* **2**, 343–57.

McCulloch, J. (1983) *Black Soul, White Artifact: Fanon's Clinical Psychology and Social Theory.* Cambridge: Cambridge University Press.

Mezzina, R. (2005) Paradigm shift in psychiatry: processes and outcomes. In S. Ramon and J.E. Williams (eds) *Mental Health at the Crossroads: The Promise of the Psychosocial Approach.* Aldershot: Ashgate, pp. 81–93.

Molnar, S. (1983) *Human Variation: Races, Types and Ethnic Groups* (2nd edn). Englewood Cliffs, NJ: Prentice-Hall.

Morel, B.-A. (1852) *Traité des Mentales.* Paris: Masson. In I.I. Gottesman, *Schizophrenia Genesis: The Origins of Madness,* New York and Oxford: Freeman, 1991.

Obeyesekere, G. (1977) The theory and practice of psychological medicine in the Ayurvedic tradition. *Culture, Medicine and Psychiatry,* **1**, 155–81.

Obeyesekere, G. (1985) Depression, Buddhism, and the work of culture in Sri Lanka. In A. Kleinman and B. Good (eds) *Culture and Depression.* Berkeley: University of California Press, pp. 134–52.

Offer, D. and Sabshin, M. (1966) *Normality: Theoretical and Clinical Concepts of Mental Health.* New York: Basic Books.

Omi, M. and Winant, H. (1994) Racial formation. In M. Omi and H. Winant (eds) *Racial Formation in the United States: From the Sixties to the Nineties* (2nd edn). New York and London: Routledge.

Pick, D. (1989) *Faces of Degeneration. A European Disorder. c.1848–c.1918.* Cambridge: Cambridge University Press.

Pieterse, J.N. (1992) *White on Black: Images of Africa and Blacks in western Culture.* New Haven, CT: Yale University Press.

Prince, R. (1968) The changing picture of depressive syndromes in Africa. *Canadian Journal of African Studies,* **1**, 177–92.

Ramon, S. and Williams, J.E. (eds) (2005) *Mental Health at the Crossroads: The Promise of the Psychosocial Approach.* Aldershot: Ashgate.

Richardson, J. and Lambert, J. (1985) *The Sociology of Race.* Ormskirk, Lancs: Causeway Press.

Said, E.W. (1994) *Culture and Imperialism.* London: Vintage.

Schwartz, M.A. and Wiggins, O.P. (1987) Typifications: the first step for clinical diagnosis in psychiatry. *Journal of Nervous and Mental Disease*, **175**, 65–77.

Singer, K. (1975) Depressive disorders from a transcultural perspective. *Social Science and Medicine*, **9**, 289–301.

Sproston, K. and Nazroo, J. (eds) (2002) *Ethnic Minority Psychiatric Illness Rates in the Community (EMPIRIC)*. London: Stationery Office.

Summerfield, D. (2001) The invention of post-traumatic stress disorder and the social usefulness of a psychiatric category. *British Medical Journal*, **322**, 95–8.

Thomas, A. and Sillen, S. (1972) *Racism and Psychiatry*. New York: Brunner/Mazel.

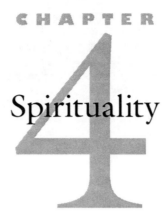

Spirituality

Phil Barker and Poppy Buchanan-Barker

BRIEF CHAPTER OUTLINE

The afterthought of the authors is presented first to help provide a context for which the chapter examines spirituality. This frame of reference enables a flow into a discussion regarding the actual experience of human 'being' and how this cannot be articulated or fully understood. Spirituality occupies this very space and asks the complex question: who are you? A number of testimonies are presented as an attempt to engage with the subject. This is followed by a brief look at 'wholeness' and the pursuit of enlightenment. The spiritual journey through this text of finding oneself, living with oneself and overcoming oneself is concluded through the coming home.

Afterthought

We break with tradition here, by reflecting on our writing of this chapter. Perhaps this irregular epilogue will provide a frame of reference for the chapter, setting it firmly within the context of our 'lived experience'.

We had written about spirituality before (Barker and Buchanan-Barker, 2004), and much of our work, especially over the past decade, had focused on what might be called the 'spirit' of the person in distress. Despite our familiarity with, or attraction to, 'spirit' we approached this chapter with some trepidation. Maybe we knew ourselves, too well, or maybe we felt awestruck by the topic. Perhaps we appreciated the problems associated with claiming to understand *what* spirituality *is*, far less what this might *mean* in a mental health context. We were aware at the outset that by the end of the chapter, *all* would certainly not be revealed, but something would undoubtedly be clearer. What that might be only time would tell.

We wrestled with these 'perhaps' and 'maybes' over an unusually hot, dry Scottish summer. In the mornings we stayed indoors to write and spent the rest of the day reopening a 'lost garden' that had been overgrown for almost a century. As the chapter began to take shape, so too did a slippery descent through the lost, cliffside garden, down to the estuary's rocky foreshore. Each day, we flitted between the dumb glare of the computer screen and the lively, flickering sun on the rippling tide.

Tapping computer keys and thrashing with sickle and shears could hardly be more different forms of work. As the days and weeks passed, however, the two seemed to fuse. We 'lost' ourselves in these labours, 'finding' ourselves only when we stood up to stretch, or wiped sweat from our brows. We were aware of feeling and thinking less and *doing* more. We were becoming, not quite effortlessly, 'the work'; letting go our usual grasp of 'me' or 'I'; those laboured, overwrought and unduly precious notions of what it means to be a person; blending into the tumbling flow of words and the swaying, chirping natural world that wrapped around 'us'...

As we worked our way carefully down the cliff, clearing ivy, nettles and countless other shrubs and weeds, we realized the symbolism of our sweaty labour. We were clambering down the cliff to reach the water, from which all life had first clambered. *Why* we were reclaiming that long-lost cliffside garden was not at all clear. Indeed, this work was no more purposeful than the writing of this chapter; both took shape, as different things were revealed, usually more by accident than design.

One afternoon, reading Thomas Moore for respite, a meaning leapt, unannounced, and refreshingly accidental, from the page.

> You have (the) capacity within you to be the poet to your experience. You have to learn how to 'sum up' your experience in images that convey your personal truth. I do it by writing books on subjects that I wrestle with personally. Many people write songs, poems, and stories. Some, less obviously, make gardens.
>
> (Moore, 2004: 9)

Were we 'conveying a personal truth' through our garden labours? Was that our intention? Or were we 'expressing' something much simpler? Who knows? We have lost track of the 'reason' why we agreed to write this chapter; and have lost touch with the spark of motivation that began our garden project. Such 'losses' are all too typical. We find ourselves, more often than not, caught up in the *flow* of time and its repetitive, changeable tides; immersed in *doing* what needs to be done: letting go of some of the incessant chatter of our minds;

becoming more 'at one' with life – and *living* – that is *purposeful* activity. However, the riddle remains: how to 'know your purpose'.

In religious terms 'atonement' means more than making up for wrongdoing or sinfulness, but means 'reconciliation with God'. This spiritual idea of 'at-one-ment' is threaded through this chapter. For us, spirituality involves a *reconnection*, if not 'reconciliation', between our isolated and sometimes fragmented 'selves', and the countless aspects of life that flow through us and around us. For some people such forces are the Hand of God (of any religion), while for others they suggest Gaia, or Mother Earth (Lovelock, 1995). Although the scientist might appear to deny the existence of any 'godhead', the physical mystery of contemporary science's 'multiple universes', and their putative 'origins', bear a striking resemblance to religious thought – merely described differently. Whether we talk of Christianity, Wicca or astrophysics, humankind is an insignificant speck in a much bigger picture. Spirituality involves recognizing our insignificance. In so doing, we heal the artificial separation between 'us' and that 'bigger picture'; becoming 'at one' with our God (however named) *or* the universe from which we emerged, and to which we shall, at some point, return.

Spirituality: meanings and metaphors

Our 'lost garden' story might seem like a rather obvious, biblical allusion, but its historical truth, not to mention the revelation of a personal truth, symbolized by our garden work, signals the importance of metaphor in the meaning of spirituality. Metaphorical meanings, and the personal and shared human values to which they are attached, appear central to the 're-emergence' of spirituality in the contemporary mental health field.

Spirituality has, only slowly, established a place within twenty-first-century mental health discourse. Dedicated 'interest groups' now exist within the Royal College of Psychiatrists, and the National Institute for Mental Health, England (NIMHE) and the Mental Health Foundation (NIMHE, 2003) collaborate on 'spirituality' projects. These developments represent only the tip of the spirituality iceberg (Gersten, 1997; Grof and Grof, 1990; Nelson, 1994) and are not without irony, given that 'spirit' was the original focus of traditional psychiatry. The *psyche,* which psychiatry sought to heal, was recognized as the human *soul* or *spirit,* long before it came to be known as the 'mind'. Sadly, contemporary psychiatry, and the popular public view of 'mental illness', has almost been taken over by a simplistic, and as yet still unfounded, view of mental distress as merely an indication of brain disturbance. People, as we shall see, tell a different, soulful story.

My madness, my sanity, my life

When Stephen Hawking (1998) talked about 'knowing the mind of God' he might have been playing with scientific metaphor, but was also repeating the aspirations of many a theologian or mystic. *Knowing* is an experience of our total being, something near-impossible to represent in words. Any form of *being* – in love, lost, alone or contented – may be talked *about,* but rarely do we get close to expressing the nub of the experience, at a *personal* level. That is the trouble with experience: we know we are having it, but as soon as we try to express the experience it falls like mercury through our clutching fingers. Asking people how they *came* to know something is as challenging as asking what *exactly* they know, and *why* they know it. We know who we are – as persons. We know we are *well,* and we know we are *ill, ailing* or *sick,* long before any doctor comes near to labelling this experience. We *know* when we experience things and we know what those experiences are. All this is easy. The problems start when we ask what this might mean, and especially when we try to explain this experience to others, who frequently leap to an 'understanding'.

Mental health workers – from all disciplines – feign such understanding. People describing themselves as 'service users', 'psychiatric survivors' or, in today's new parlance, 'experts by experience', do likewise, often talking as if they have a special gift for understanding *and* representing others, described as 'mentally ill'. Can one person who has lost the will to live speak for *everyone* who has contemplated suicide? Can one person who has felt anxious and alienated speak for everyone who has felt the world crashing in upon them? Madness is such a variegated, encyclopaedic, and at the same time highly personal form of human being that it is genuine folly to suggest that one person could fully understand and represent the experiences of another. The bald truth is that *everyone* is an 'expert': but only on their own experience. Life is absolute. People may *relate* to another's experience, believing that they are in full *empathy* with their experience, but this is only superficial. More often than not this affinity is illusory.

> No one can live it (my life) for me. No one can serve it for me. My work, my suffering, my joy, are absolute. There's no way, for instance, you can feel the pain in my toe; or I can feel the pain in your toe. You can't sleep for me. You can't swallow for me. And that is the paradox: in totally owning the pain, the joy, the responsibility of my life – if I see this point clearly – then I'm free. I have no hope, I have no need for anything else.
>
> (Beck, 1997: 65)

Beck's view is necessarily provocative. *Hope* is increasingly seen as an important part of mental health services, especially those with a 'holistic', 'spiritual' or recovery focus (e.g. NIMHE, 2003). Charlotte Joko Beck, the Zen teacher, expresses here one of *her* 'personal truths' about life. What she believes, or has found to be 'true', rings a loud bell with us but clashes head-on with the contemporary 'hopeful' mental health rhetoric.

> Joko has little patience with romanticised spirituality, idealized 'sweetness and light' that seeks to bypass reality and the suffering it brings. She is fond of quoting a line from the *Shoyu Roku:* 'From the withered tree, a flower blooms'. Through living each moment as it is, the ego gradually drops away, revealing the wonder of everyday life.
>
> (Smith, 1997: ix)

If we are genuinely *curious* about life – that which we call 'our own' and all other forms of life that we encounter – we have no need for hope. A powerful firebird will rise from the ashes of our miserable experience. The more terrifying the darkness, the more it will illuminate the faintest glimmer of light. *Hope* will only get in the way, encouraging us to struggle and strive, expecting something other than that which is right in front of our noses. Beck adds a view, which speaks directly to the field of 'mental health' – especially the 'self-development' or 'personal growth' areas.

> We are usually living in vain hope for something or someone that will make *my* life easier, more pleasant. We spend most of our time trying to set up life in a way so that it will be true; when, contrariwise, the joy of life is just in totally doing and just bearing what must be borne, in just doing what has to be done. It's not even what *has* to be done; its there to be done so we do it.
>
> (Beck, 1997: 65)

Contemporary psychiatry and psychology are a world away from this paradoxical view. With their scientific pretensions, intent on *explaining* human experience, many mental health practitioners claim to 'know' what is happening for people, or more impertinently, to know 'what's *really* happening'; assuming to understand what this *means*. Usually, this is just a preamble to the offer of a solution, remedy or other corrective for the ailing 'spirit'. *Hope* may feature nowadays in mental health literature, especially internet websites, but usually this is restricted to 'hope' for a 'correct diagnosis' and 'appropriate treatment'.

We can offer only *our* understanding of other people's stories. We *cannot* ever know the truth of their story. Such humility is vital if we are to avoid controlling, containing or otherwise pigeonholing the sublimely personal nature of experience. The simple truth of spirituality is that people have all that they need to embark on and explore the spiritual dimension of their lives, in the same way that they are ideally equipped to come to an understanding, of everything else associated with their personal experience. Everything else – this chapter included – is merely a commercial enterprise: promoting someone else's ideas, theory or philosophy.

Regrettably, some people live out long lives but seem to have few 'experiences', at least as we understand them. Instead, they follow 'life scripts' (Steiner, 1990) echoing the experience of others, or otherwise fitting in with the social and cultural mores of the day. For some people madness may be a thickly disguised 'wake-up call', challenging the person to 'get real', to awaken to all the joy and suffering that life has to offer. Young people frequently complain of 'being bored', since 'nothing ever happens here'. Many adults carry this blinkered outlook throughout their lives, failing to appreciate the wonder of existence, although not necessarily 'wonderful' as the word is commonly understood. What used to be called 'the neuroses' takes this miserly outlook to an extreme. People complain about experiences, asking others to do something to help it 'go away', or otherwise make life more 'pleasant'. Maybe our current depression epidemic is an offshoot from the great Urge to Happiness, and the Obsession with Novelty, which has dominated western culture for the past 30 years. The pursuit of Self, and its improvement, coupled with our desire to 'enhance' the body, are all unashamedly cosmetic: covering the 'who' of the person with layers of image. Such is the packaged self – all surface, no content.

The name is not the thing

People may not know – in any definitive sense – what has upset their lives, or otherwise ails them, but attributing this to the disturbing effects of *biochemistry* (biological), *dysfunctional belief systems* (psychological), *childhood upbringing* (social) or all three (biopsychosocial) is not far removed from talking about possession by demons – still frowned upon when reported in 'primitive' cultures. Contemporary scientific 'explanations' are seen by many to reduce stigma, showing that the person is not responsible for their troubles. However, people don't invite 'demons' either, so where does that leave us?

Most of the changes in the madness industry over the past half-century have been linguistic. In the 1950s, over 100 forms of madness were 'classified'. Today there are close on 400. In a categorical sense, we are now four times as crazy as 50 years ago (Kirk and Kutchins, 1997). Spirituality sidesteps the lunacy of diagnosis, which may be part of its contemporary appeal. Spirituality also echoes poetry, literature, opera and the visual arts, if not also magic, ritual and humanity's primeval relationship with time and place, where the mystery of life is documented and detailed, but never 'explained'. It is easy to talk about spirituality in the arts or when describing the Aboriginal 'Dreamtime' (Voigt and Drury, 1997) or the mental health problems of 'Muslim communities' in multicultural Britain (James, 2005). However, when spoken aloud in public, or expressed in print, spirituality can trigger some powerful resistance, especially for its assumed relationship with organized religion, or worse, for its association with the wackier aspects of the New Age. The critic will ask, if 'mental illness' is a function of a 'chemical imbalance', then why are we meditating, chanting, burning incense, or (worse) trying to make sense of it? From a medical, scientific, statistical, economic point of view, this is a reasonable question.

Spirituality occupies a different, and quite awkward space. How might one 'show' that spirituality was 'useful'? Many marriages end in divorce. Does this mean that 'marriage' doesn't work or is no longer 'useful'? What do we mean by 'work' or 'useful' anyway? As they stand, these are daft questions.

In the 'mental health' context, spirituality seems to be about journey and exploration, and may even be far away from anything as straightforward as 'understanding'. The 'spiritual' is the antithesis of rationality. Instead of reassuring us with logic, spirituality impersonates Scrooge's ghostly Christmas visitors: beckoning us to look beyond the veneer of our lives; rummaging through the tidy, ordered personal, social and cultural borders of our lives. The diagnostician says we are 'psychotic' or 'clinically depressed'. We ask ourselves: what does this mean? What is this all about? Why this? Why now? The more adventurous spirit might ask: What is Life trying to tell me? At its most extreme, spirituality seems to ask the simplest yet, paradoxically, most complex, question: Who *are* you?

Testimonies

Brian Wilson was hailed as a musical genius in the 1960s but became, less than a decade later, part of the huge catalogue of remarkable literary, musical, artistic and scientific figures viewed, in their day as a 'mad genius' (Barker, 1998). Even in the USA, where therapy was a way of life, Wilson went beyond the pale – becoming an embarrassment to his fellow Beach Boys. He gradually slipped into what he later described as a spiritual abyss but, with support, slowly climbed back up into the sunshine. In his autobiography, he described his entry into 'the dark night of the soul' first described, poetically, by Juan de la Cruz (St John of the Cross, 1542–91). Finding himself on a deserted beach, feeling suicidal, he wrestled with the inconsistencies of his life. How could he write beautiful music that enchanted millions, but still suffer confusion and inner torment?

> Feeling shipwrecked on an existential island, I lost myself in the blanket of darkness that stretched beyond the breaking waves to the other side of the Earth. The ocean so vast, the universe so large, and suddenly I saw myself in proportion to that, a little pebble of sand, a jellyfish floating on top of the water, travelling with the current. I felt dwarfed, temporary.
>
> (Wilson, 1993: 193–4)

That seaside epiphany marked the start of Brian Wilson's 20-year-long recovery of himself and the meaning of his life. Like many others with deep personal crises, the blinding light of revelation was pretty ordinary, but the recovery journey it signalled was long and arduous. But, like everyone who sees the light, however flickering, the experience was full of meaning. What, exactly, did Brian Wilson 'find' or begin to realize, as he wrestled, metaphorically, with himself and aspects of his life?

Sally Clay shuttled in and out of psychiatric hospitals for over 30 years. Although a Buddhist, she set her own spiritual struggle in a biblical context:

> Jacob named the place of his struggle Peniel, which means 'face of God'. I too have seen God face to face and I want to remember my Peniel. I really do not want to be recovered. From the experience of madness I received a wound that changed my life. It enabled me to help others and to know myself. I am proud that I have struggled with God and with the mental health system. I have not recovered. I have overcome.
>
> (Clay, 1999)

Brian Wilson may be a tormented genius – like William Blake or Tchaikovsky – and Sally Clay may be something of a mystic – like Teresa of Avila or C.S. Lewis. Both remind us that for each celebrity who steps 'into the mystic' (as Van Morrison said), there exist hundreds of similar, but unsung, spiritual travellers among the so-called 'mentally ill'. Not to say that *all* madness has a spiritual basis, or that all people with 'mental health problems' want to explore their spirituality. However, lots of people who have been pushed to the farthest reaches of their own human nature have slowly begun to make sense of the experience. Like characters from mythology, they wrestled with their demons and became the heroes of their own stories.

Spirituality involves connecting with the bigger picture, locating our tiny selves in the greater whole. The spirit is often defined negatively, in terms of everything that is *not* material or physical. We 'admire someone's spirit' but are hard pressed to say, exactly, *what* this is. The 'spiritual' is something we *know*, deep within ourselves. When asked to define such 'knowledge', words fail us. This explains why we turn to poetry, music, or art to express, symbolically, what Van Morrison called *'the inarticulate speech of the heart'* (Hinton, 2003).

Spirituality is often confused with religion. All faiths have spiritual origins but customs and rituals often dominate organized religion. For some, religion is simply the form spirituality takes in a specific civilization (Thompson, 1981). By contrast, spiritual experiences are often highly personal – often lacking any sense of order. As such, they can be threatening – as Brian Wilson and Sally Clay showed. This suggests something of the power that lies beyond our everyday selves. This might signal God, the Absolute, or the Cosmos; or perhaps is just a sign of our own latent power, waiting to come to life. The *epiphany* – or realization – associated with deep spiritual encounters, is a 'wake-up call'. Something significant has happened and nothing will ever be the same again.

People with experience of psychosis frequently talk about the personal meanings of their 'breakdowns' (Barker, Campbell and Davidson, 1999), many describing this as part of a spiritual journey. Their spiritual wake-up calls seemed to have been forced by the breakdown itself. The terror and confusion of madness seemed to be a necessary evil: something they had to go through to find meaning in life, echoing Buddha's invitation to follow their own path to spiritual understanding: 'Be ye lamps unto yourselves, be your own reliance. Hold on to the truth within yourselves, as to the only lamp' (Goddard, 1956).

Our friend, the New Zealand poet and mental health advocate, Gary Platz, was a window cleaner. One day, the sun temporarily blinded him and he realized that he was 'the Redeemer'. In time, he came to realize that it was himself who needed redemption. By then, he had a psychotic diagnosis, and had discovered how psychiatric treatment invalidated *all* of his experiences, not just his spiritual side. Gary wrote:

> Who am I to say who I am?
> When I'm told my brain isn't right
> And people give it names
> Which take away mine.
> *Yes this stigma acid eats my soul.*
> (Platz, 2004)

The struggle to reclaim his voice and human identity was central to Gary's recovery. 'For me spirituality wasn't a factor in recovery from madness towards some form of sanity. Rather, madness was essential in the recovery process from a spiritual crisis' (p. 201).

One night Peter Wilkin was asked to 'special' a suicidal man. As he sat at his bedside he was struck by a realization:

> He turned towards me, eyes closed...and gripped the bedclothes tightly in his hand...blankets too rough for comfort. I saw his face and smelled his rank odour...I was his sentinel – yet sat in his dungeon. He was the one with needles in his eyes, so desperate to jump from his mortal coil. Yet it was I – in the black hole of my yawning insignificance – who heard the death knell ringing.
>
> (Wilkin, 2004: 160)

These testimonies show people confronting their insignificance and, paradoxically, realising their sublime importance, as part of the 'bigger picture'. Being alive, as a human being, offers a precious opportunity. We are no more than a drop in the ocean of eternal life, or are simply a grain of sand, picked up from all the grains on the shores of life. We are unique yet also connected to the whole.

One of the tragedies of life is when we fail to appreciate how precious is the gift of life, with all the joy and misery that accompanies it. Having been given human life – *being* that identifiable droplet from the ocean or grain from the beach – we need nothing more. When we experience our spirit, we realise that 'all hope is about sizing up the past and projecting it into the future' (Beck, 1997: 63). When we find (and lose) ourselves *in the moment* we realize that 'there is no past and no future except in our minds. There is nothing but self and self always is here, present...We hope for something that's going to take care of this little self because we don't realise that already we are self. There's nothing around us that is not self. What are we looking for?' (Beck, 1997: 63).

Despite all our twenty-first-century sophistication, we remain in the grip of a Cartesian worldview: still believing that because 'I think *therefore* I am', still trying to construct a split, or separation, between *who* we are and *what* we experience. A simpler, yet more complex, notion of self is that 'I *am*'. When 'I' eat or drink or laugh or cry, 'I' is to be found in these acts of eating, drinking, laughing or crying. Where else could 'I' be? Our pursuit of 'self-consciousness' and 'self-awareness' is deeply flawed. Making his own connection, 40 years ago, between Christian and Zen 'consciousness', Thomas Merton summarized our flawed ambition thus:

> Modern man...is a subject for whom his self-awareness as a thinking, observing, measuring and estimating 'self' is absolutely primary. The more he is able to develop his consciousness as a subject over against objects, the more he can understand things in their relations to him and one another, the more he can manipulate these objects for his own interests, but also, at the same time, the more he tends to isolate himself in his own subjective prison, to become a detached observer cut off from everything else in a kind of impenetrable alienated and transparent bubble, which contains all reality in the form of purely subjective experience. Modern consciousness then tends to create this solipsistic bubble of awareness – an ego-self imprisoned in its own consciousness, isolated and out of touch with other such selves in so far as they are all 'things' rather than persons.
>
> (Merton, [1968] 1986: 129–30)

Helping one another towards wholeness

Many of the great 'success' stories in contemporary mental health involve people 'coming together', bonding, connecting, if not actually living with and for one another. Some such communities have a dedicated religious core, like *Alcoholics Anonymous*, but might equally simply band around a common experience, as in the *Hearing Voices Network*, various 'mutual support groups', or supported 'self-help' groups like Grow (www.grow.ie). A common feature of such groups is to 'bear witness', or give 'testimony' in different ways, sharing their experience with others, finding or making connections. Often, given the perplexing nature of such experiences, people may tell their story lyrically – as in Survivor's Poetry (www.survivorspoetry.com) – or through some other art form, which embraces the metaphor of existence: the thing of which we cannot speak, or at least, not directly (Dax, 1998). Through sharing, in different ways, experiences of madness, people appear to remedy their sense of aloneness, but also, ironically, come to know that this is a fact of human existence.

Some forms of psychotherapy followed, perhaps unwittingly, the path recommended by the Buddha and Socrates, who both suggested the power of 'looking within': examining life as a way of revealing meaning. Indeed, understanding life may be both the beginning and end of the spiritual journey that begins in psychotherapy, but cannot be completed in such an ultimately mundane activity.

People caught in the spiral of madness often try, desperately, to return to wholeness – feeling as if they are threatened with complete disintegration. For many, this begins with self-realization and the search for meaning, exploring the states of being that appear to use the most of themselves. Rather than try to establish how the person 'became' like this, we might help the person explore what this apparent collapse and disintegration might be about: what are its hidden meanings; what is the person trying to accomplish within this spiritual crisis?

Karasu (2003) believed that material possessions, success, power and pleasure often fail to fill the void that lies at the heart of our lives. Regrettably, some only replace materialism with a search for 'enlightenment' and the life of a 'spiritual tourist' (Brown, 1998). As far as Karasu is concerned, we have no option but to begin to explore the deepest yearnings of our heart. Especially in the West, our greatest yearning may be for 'happiness' (Whiteside, 2001) but, as Karasu noted, there is no end to the journey to 'real happiness'. Indeed, there is not even a good place to start. We need to start here, where we are, to begin the journey NOW!

Coming home

For us, spirituality is a question without an answer, something we look for but do not actually expect to find. As we try to live our lives in pursuit of a higher understanding of ourselves, and our place in the universe, we examine all that we know of what is inside and outside ourselves. In our Celtic spiritual tradition, the journey we take towards understanding always leads home. The

Celtic knot symbolizes the journey – snaking outwards, it eventually loops back to where it started – the hearth of home. John O'Donohue (1997) reminded us that, although we are often told that the spiritual journey involves a sequence of stages, this is an illusion: 'You do not need to go away outside your self to come into real conversation with your soul and the mysteries of your spiritual world. The eternal is at home – within you' (O'Donohue, 1997: 120).

In New Zealand, Julie Leibrich (2001) found a similar understanding of spirituality: 'It is a kind of coming home. For me, the meaning of spirituality is meaning itself.' Leibrich's experience may well signal an important 'change of heart' in the whole field of spirituality and mental health:

> My definition of mental health has a lot in common with the way I define spirituality. Both concepts are concerned with the experience of self. One reaching into dimensions of space to discover self, the other realising the freedom that comes from accepting self. That is why spiritual experiences and their interpretation can have such a profound influence on mental health.
>
> (Leibrich, 2001)

Leibrich appreciated that there might be something 'in' the space of her Self that might ultimately be of great value.

Although spirituality is increasingly included in mental health policy, is this anything more than lip service, or worse, an unscrupulous nod towards consumerism? For most people, the experience of madness, however it is labelled, is a psychic injury, from which it is often near-impossible to recover. However, many do live fruitful lives, despite their psychic hurt. For most, the experience of mental health services is little more than insult added to injury. We are now more than 100 years into the 'scientific' era of 'modern psychiatry' and in many senses we are informed beyond our wildest imaginings. However, we still struggle to understand what madness might mean for the people so afflicted, demonized and tormented.

Spirituality does not promise any 'quick fix' for the meaninglessness of contemporary practice, but it might point us back to the person – the overflowing reservoir of knowledge and potential understanding of whatever is going on under the storm clouds of madness (Culliford, 2002). All we need do is go and ask. But first we must gird our own 'spiritual' loins in preparation for what the person's story might mean for us. For the simple truth is that we are not alone – only disconnected.

The necessarily vague concept of spirituality has been endorsed, as noted already, by the government-funded National Institute for Mental Health England (NIMHE, 2003). This group aims to *'produce a policy guidance document on the value of spirituality in mental health'* and to *'broaden the understanding of clinical outcomes so as to include user goals'*. The bureaucratic language illustrates another risk – death by assimilation. Like other powerful human experiences – love, loyalty, faith or purpose – spirituality is beyond words. To define it, explain it and predict its value is to risk killing it: like telling an audience *why* a joke is funny. Nobody laughs. We already know the value of spirituality in mental health (McMullen, 2003; Zohar and Marshall, 2001). Do we really need research studies and policies, which will only turn it into another 'product' or 'process'?

Much contemporary mental health care promises quick-fix solutions, encouraging people to believe, for instance, that a short course of programmatic therapy, such as a dozen sessions of CBT, offers a cure-all. If only it was that simple. There is now a genuine risk that mental health services will build into their 'standards' some kind of Mickey-Mouse 'spirituality', sweetening the bitter pill that we all have to swallow if we are to learn the lessons that life presents to us.

Some will see this as a stoical, if not masochistic outlook on life, when it is only a realistic one. Many people spend vast portions of their waking day dreaming or hoping for 'something better', usually rendered through the old complaint: 'There has to be more to life than this!' As they devote hours, days, weeks and eventually years of their lives to such hopeful aspiration – for a glamorous partner, a well-toned body, a straighter nose, a more satisfying job that also pays better – they fail to appreciate what life has placed directly in front of them. Invariably, this results in them simply going through the motions of living, half-asleep.

Life can be lived passionately, even if *all* we are doing is sweeping leaves, ringing tills or helping people to use the toilet. Anything that *needs* doing needs to be done carefully, with our full attention. This is so simple that it becomes, again paradoxically, one of the hardest things we can ever do in life. By *taking care* as we speak – weighing our words carefully, picking up meanings from others carefully – we lose our isolated, disconnected selves *in* conversation. By *taking care* as we work, we lose ourselves in the challenge of the task, however simple or complex it might be, becoming *at one* with the act itself.

This is how we work our way through life, dissolving our fragile ego-self in the act of living. For the Buddhist, the flawed sense that we are the centre of the universe slips, effortlessly, into the Void, as we become at one with our labours. For the Christian, we let go of our vanity and God works through us, taking up residence in us, and us in Him. All of this easy to do, in principle, but requires a lifetime of daily practice to realize.

Simone Weil wrote about the apprentice who, when hurt or complaining of tiredness, is told by the other workmen that, finally, 'the trade is entering his body'.

> Each time we have some pain to go through, we can say to ourselves quite truly that it is the universe, the order, and beauty of the world and the obedience of creation to God that are entering our body. After that how can we fail to bless with tenderest gratitude the Love that sends us this gift?
>
> (Weil, 1951)

Both madness and spiritual encounters reconnect us with the core of our human being. The words are different but the experiences can be very similar. Out of chaos, we may discover order. Out of conflict we may find peace. But we need support to make such vital sense of our experience.

═══════════ **EDITORS' QUESTIONS** ═══════════

Issues of difference

■ Are there gender differences in the experience of spirituality?

■ How does sexual orientation influence the experience of spirituality?

■ What cultural differences might there be in a spiritual crisis?

Relevance to practice

■ How do mental health professionals communicate spiritual concern for a service user?

■ Can spiritual needs be assessed?

■ How do you consider and acknowledge the person's journey?

Investigate

■ What does spiritual mean to you?

■ How does your team advocate for those too vulnerable to explain their spiritual position?

■ Who are you?

Suggested further reading

Barker, P. and Buchanan-Barker, P. (eds) (2004) *Spirituality and Mental Health: Breakthrough.* London: Whurr.

Brown, M. (1998*) The Spiritual Tourist: A Personal Odyssey Through the Outer Reaches of Belief.* London: Bloomsbury.

References

Barker, P. (1998) Creativity and psychic distress in writers, artists and scientists. *Journal of Psychiatric and Mental Health Nursing* 5(2) 109–18.

Barker, P. and Buchanan-Barker, P. (eds) (2004) *Spirituality and Mental Health: Breakthrough.* London: Whurr.

Barker, P., Campbell, P. and Davidson, B. (1999) *From the Ashes of Experience: Reflections on Madness, Survival and Growth.* London: Whurr.

Beck, C.J. (1997*) Everyday Zen: Love and Work.* London: Thorsons.

Brown, M. (1998*), The Spiritual Tourist: A Personal Odyssey Through the Outer Reaches of Belief.* London: Bloomsbury.

Clay, S. (1999), Madness and reality. In P. Barker, P. Campbell and B. Davidson (eds) *From the Ashes of Experience: Reflections on Madness, Recovery and Growth.* London: Whurr.

Culliford, L. (2002) Spiritual care and psychiatric treatment: an introduction. *Advances in Psychiatric Treatment* 8, 249–61.

Dax, E.C. (1998) *The Cunningham Dax Collection: Selected Works of Psychiatric Art.* Melbourne: Melbourne University Press.

Gersten, D. (1997) *Are You Getting Enlightened or Losing Your Mind?* New York: Random House.

Goddard, D. (1956) *A Buddhist Bible.* London: Harrap.

Grof, S. and Grof, C. (1990) *The Stormy Search for Self.* Los Angeles: Tarcher.

Hawking, S. (1998) *A Brief History of Time.* London: Bantam.

Hinton, B. (2003) *Celtic Crossroads: The Art of Van Morrison.* London: Sanctuary.

James, A. (2005) A voice in the wilderness. *Guardian,* 25 June.

Karasu, T.B. (2003) *The Art of Serenity.* New York: Simon & Schuster.

Kirk, S.A. and Kutchins, H. (1997) *Making us Crazy: The Psychiatric Bible and the Creation of Mental Disorders.* New York: Free Press.

Leibrich, J. (2001) *Making Space: Spirituality and Mental Health.* Mary Hemingway Rees Memorial Lecture, World Assembly for Mental Health, Vancouver, July.

Lovelock, J. (1995) *The Ages of Gaia: A Biography of Our Living Earth.* New York: Norton.

McMullen, B. (2003) Spiritual intelligence. *British Medical Journal Career Focus* **326**: S51.

Merton, T. ([1968] 1986) *Zen and the Birds of Appetite.* New York: New Directions. Reprinted in John Garvey (ed.) *Modern Spirituality: An Anthology.* London: Darton, Longman & Todd.

Moore, T. (2004) *Dark Nights of the Soul.* London: Piatkus.

Nelson, J.E. (1994) *Healing the Split: Integrating Spirit into our Understanding of the Mentally Ill.* Albany, New York: State University of New York Press.

NIMHE (2003) *Inspiring Hope: Recognising the Importance of Spirituality in a Whole-Person Approach to Mental Health.* Leeds: National Institute for Mental Health, England.

O'Donohue, J. (1997) *Anam Cara: Spiritual Wisdom from the Celtic World.* London: Bantam.

Platz, G. (2004) Spirituality, madness and the man who lost a thousand masks. In P. Barker. and P. Buchanan-Barker (eds) *Spirituality and Mental Health: Breakthrough.* London: Whurr, p. 203.

Smith, S. (1997) Preface. In C.J. Beck, *Everyday Zen: Love and Work.* London: Thorsons.

Steiner, C.M. (1990) *Scripts People Live: Transactional Analysis of Life Scripts* (2nd edn). New York: Grove Press.

Thompson, W.I. (1981) *The Time Falling Bodies Take to Light: Mythology, Sexuality and the Origins of Culture.* New York: St Martin's Press/Praeger.

Voigt, A. and Drury, N. (1997) *Wisdom of the Earth: The Living Legacy of the Aboriginal Dreamtime.* East Roseville, NSW, Australia: Simon & Schuster.

Weil, S. (1951) *Waiting for God.* New York, Putnam. Reprinted in John Garvey (ed.) *Modern Spirituality: An Anthology.* London: Darton, Longman & Todd, 1986.

Whiteside, P. (2001), *Happiness: The 30-day Guide.* London: Rider Books.

Wilkin, P. (2004) *Epiphanies.* In P. Barker and P. Buchanan-Barker (eds) *Spirituality and Mental Health: Breakthrough.* London: Whurr, p. 160.

Wilson, B. (1993) *Wouldn't it be Nice: My Own Story.* London: Bloomsbury.

Zohar, D. and Marshall, I. (2001) *SQ: The Ultimate Intelligence.* London: Bloomsbury.

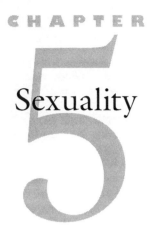

CHAPTER

5

Sexuality

Robert Tummey and David T. Evans

BRIEF CHAPTER OUTLINE

Sexuality is explored here through the perspective of three main concepts, noted by the World Health Organization. First, the chapter considers the place of sexuality within the lifespan and being central to human life. From childhood, through adulthood and then older adulthood, a variety of aspects are discussed, such as age of consent, sexuality as core identity and the right of sexual expression. The next section explores how sexuality is experienced and expressed, contributing to mental distress. Then, sexuality influenced by interaction is highlighted. This incorporates the impact of mental illness and care on sexuality, with a need for responsible policy making and mature acknowledgement of sexual need by mental health services. The chapter concludes with ways to move forward.

Introduction

The concept of sexuality and mental health poses quite a challenge in health care and society. Both bring about judgements and strong opinion. Both can involve the deep value-systems that can often be constructed as taboo and primarily addressed through an everyday language of euphemistic stereotypy. With such influence on perception, it is of interest that the subject is rarely discussed in mental health care, seemingly confined to misunderstood denial or even worse, nonexistence. Sexuality encompasses many things to different people, including expression, orientation, status, identity and the actual mechanics of sex. With such a cloak of taboo surrounding it, sexuality is filled with intrigue and worthy of further exploration.

During the 1980s it was apparent that western societies became hooked on all things sexual (as discussed by Greer, 1984 and Heath, 1982) to the extent that for some commentators, sexuality became the prime medium through which people 'define their personalities...establish their identities...become conscious of themselves' (Foucault and Sennett, 1981: 22). This new-found revolution transformed the way in which society views the sexual status of the individual or group, but not for people with mental illness. The perception of their asexual status has remained unchanged. No such liberation or freedom of their sexuality can be seen or identified throughout this so-called sexual revolution.

A number of issues surrounding sexuality and mental health deserve attention, but space requires a selection that is in keeping with the nature of this book. While sexual status may have been liberated, the debate on sexuality and sexual expression is a subject that remains taboo in society. People working in mental health care are a product of their society and bring with them the attitude, prejudice, sexual discrimination and boundaries of the perceived norms for behaviour. In an attempt to provide some guidance on the subject and consider what sexuality and expression actually is, a working definition was elaborated as a result of a World Health Organization International Consultation on sexual health in January 2002. It determined that:

- Sexuality is a central aspect of being human throughout life and encompasses sex, gender identities and roles, sexual orientation, eroticism, pleasure, intimacy and reproduction.

- Sexuality is experienced and expressed in thoughts, fantasies, desires, beliefs, attitudes, values, behaviours, practices, roles and relationships.

- Sexuality is influenced by the interaction of biological, psychological, social, economic, political, cultural, ethical, legal, historical, religious and spiritual factors.

(WHO, Gender and Reproductive Rights:
http://www.who.int/reproductive-health/
gender/sexual_health.html) [accessed 03/02/08]

For the purpose of this chapter, the WHO working definition will form the structure through which the subject will be explored. By no means will this chapter be a definitive guide on sexuality for the mental health practitioner. It will, however, provide some insight into the difficulties, stigma, shame and confusion experienced by people regarding their sexuality and how that influences their mental health. Also, to explore how mental health care influences the opportunity, expression and attitude to sexuality, through the institution and treatment offered. Throughout this chapter a candid view will determine the current situation, the influences and the provocative. Sexuality in mental health care will be explored, and consideration for the diversity of sexual need, orientation and gratification. The subject of sexual abuse has been purposefully avoided. This is a separate topic, albeit related.

Sexuality as central to human life

Childhood and sexuality

Our earliest schooling and peer-group play establish the fundamental characteristics of 'natural' male and female gender and 'sexual' difference through slang labels such as, 'slut', 'tart' 'whore,' 'queer', 'poof' and 'dyke' (see Lees, 1993; Mac an Ghail, 1994), which serve as key normative warning signposts, even before we fully know what they mean. They signify that sexual identity is at the very core of contemporary social life; that there are severely stigmatized sexual statuses to be ashamed of, and if we can't avoid them we should at least carefully conceal them for fear of name-calling and weightier sanctions such as ridicule, bullying and physical attack. Indeed, our learning of these terms in our most formative years, alongside early physical explorations in peer-group play beyond the parental gaze, establishes a lifelong fixation on sexuality as an obsession with something dark, deeply private, mysterious, threatening and secretive (Gagnon, 1967). Thereafter common-sense negotiations with the meanings of sexuality maintain this 'secret' either by defusing the seriousness of sexuality and its related mental health problems, or asserting its inexplicability through references to the mysteries of 'attraction', 'love' and 'romance'.

The language of sexuality and childhood becomes the language of disputed rights. For example, the sex education of children, their access to 'sexual' health care, contraception and abortion are fraught with tensions and conflicts over parental, children's, health-care workers' and teachers' rights and responsibilities; leading to simple avoidance, ignorance, confusion and distress. In the UK 'children' and 'childhood' are vigorously protected by the state and law on grounds of their assumed natural 'asexuality' or 'innocence', yet within a wider context in which they are increasingly 'sexualized' by marketing strategies and practices, whether it be through fashion, pop music or, increasingly, cosmetic surgery. Oddly, such paradoxes and their related 'mental health' implications are rarely picked up in the reported ruminations of medical researchers who consistently detach sexuality from the materialist contexts in which it is constructed and exploited.

Children at present receive very little education about sexuality, from the point of view of rights, expression, consent, infections/diseases, actual mechanics, emotional attachment, gender difference in experience, loving sex, abuse, gaining further knowledge and so on. In a recent survey by Childline, the 24-hour children's helpline run by NSPCC in the UK, it was found that over four-fifths of parents of school-age children (83 per cent) think schools should teach young people about emotional aspects of sex and relationships as well as the biological facts. They also highlighted that children calling the helpline feel pressure to have sex at an early age, but lack knowledge about sexual health, staying safe and contraception. Childline are calling for the government to review personal, social and health education (PSHE) to include learning about sexuality, relationships, safe sex and pregnancy and to make this a statutory requirement in England (Mental Health Foundation, 2006).

When considering the sexual citizenship, rights and maturity of childhood sexuality it is interesting to determine the legal age of consent to sex across the world. The UK has set the age at 16 years for consent to sex for both hetero-sexuals and homosexuals. However, there is international disparity and vari-ation in the ages of consent to sex. Here is a brief selective overview of ages to consent:

UK: 16 years for both heterosexual and homosexual sex.

Zimbabwe: male homosexual sex is illegal.

Spain, South Korea: 13 years for both heterosexual and homosexual sex.

South Africa: 16 years for heterosexual sex, 19 years for homosexual sex.

Pakistan: Must be married for heterosexual sex. Homosexual sex is illegal (this is similar across all Islamic states and a number of African countries).

USA: various ages across the States from 14 to 18 years for heterosexual sex and disparity across many states for homosexual sex, with the law repealed and invalidated (there are some states with ages from 15 to 18 years for homosexual sex).

Nigeria: 13 years for heterosexual sex and homosexual sex is illegal.

China: 14 years for both heterosexual and homosexual sex.
(Worldwide Ages of Consent: http://www.avert.org/
aofconsent.htm) [accessed 02/02/08]

This raises a number of fundamental, ethical dilemmas for the people born within a liberal or restricting environment and now living in an opposite cul-ture or legal perspective. It can apply to the very core values of an individual whose instinct may be to reject homosexuality as illegal or their acceptance of 13 as the age of consent. Mental health services will employ people from vari-ous backgrounds and countries to work with mental illness and vulnerability, so their perception of sexuality will be defined by their country of origin and may be an opposing view to the dominant legal system of their adopted country.

Adulthood and sexuality

When childhood has been navigated and the realm of adulthood is reached, the ability to express sexuality and consent to sex is one of legal, moral and cultural ease, understanding and norm. However, it is not an easy transition. Sex and sexuality are rarely discussed and norms are rarely identified. The con-cept of sexuality resides in a taboo position of mystery and secrecy. Whether heterosexual or homosexual, sexuality is a defining feature of a core identity, navigating adult norms that are to be confirmed through marriage, a relationship, cohabiting, living together and so on.

Sexuality is expressed in many ways throughout adulthood, whether subtle or obvious, loving, sensual, sexy or flirtatious. It can also be determined as deviant, perverse, bizarre, crude, disgusting or disturbing, as perceived within the boundaries of sexual norms. Yet there is a tolerance of 'so-called' deviant behaviour within the norm, through a booming sex industry that offers pornographic magazines in newsagents, DVDs available for hire, dedicated channels on cable TV, websites and so on. Indeed, even when staying in a hotel there are discreet pornographic channels to choose from. One may not choose to access these services, but it is clear that many do so.

Adults require the means to actively engage in meeting their sexual needs. This can obviously spill into illegal practice, abuse and exploitation, with mental health issues a possible consequence. Sexuality can be a celebration of being alive, an act of procreation, a loving exchange or just plain 'getting off' on the moment of intimacy with someone else or alone. But what of the impact on mental health or the impact of having mental health problems? Is sexuality considered central to the human life of people suffering from mental illness? It is suggested not. A few possible barriers are considered below:

- Social isolation
- Lack of social skills
- Lack of practice
- Lack of opportunity
- Lack of confidence
- Low self-esteem
- Negative self perception
- Perceived as deviant
- Perceived as asexual

- Shame and guilt
- Fear and retribution
- Religious influence
- Previous sexual abuse
- Side-effects of medication
- Sexual dysfunction
- Lack of education
- A solitary pursuit
- Lack of interest

It can be difficult for many people to conform to the perceived societal norm, as the following list may suggest: adultery, separation, abuse, exploitation, sex offenders, paedophiles, date rape, molestation, blurring of sexual boundaries, media sexual imagery, pornography, sex workers and so on. Therefore, is the actual norm well defined or ill-defined? The issue of sex and sexuality of people with mental illness should not be categorized against such ambiguous concepts and having their need for sexual expression demonized and pathologized into something less than natural; particularly in light of our culture's inundation with media messages about sex (Mossman, Perlin and Dorfman, 1997). Furthermore, they should be enabled to establish their own sexuality as central to their life, alongside everyone else.

Older adulthood and sexuality

Despite the overwhelming evidence of indeed now living as sexual beings in a social world dominated by sexual concerns, behaviours and identities, certain constituencies within populations and institutional settings therein are either assumed to be, or specifically defined as, non-sexual, and with an either masked or fiercely protected sexual potential. Extensive research on treatment of older adults by all agencies, but especially within nursing and care-home environments, demonstrates that individuals within are rarely defined as sexual, or, more accurately, assumed to be anything other than heterosexual, and where aspects of sexuality arise, they are defused to be avoided as far as possible (Hubbard *et al.*, 2003; Powers, 1996; Roach, 2004).

Older adults are significant because of numerical size. They are routinely defined as 'non-sexual' because they are 'not able', are economically inactive and lack consumer power. They are a perceived economic burden on the state and, in short, completely fail to make the idealized pursuit of the sexual self that drives those who are younger. Its significance extends further, of course, especially within the care-home or nursing-home context, owing to the sexual being as much a matter of mind and body, and older adults being easily dismissed for 'losing' both. In a culture in which it is assumed that all have a sexual identity, older people are no longer treated as though they still have one, or, more seriously, as though they ever had one.

Everyone is merely assumed to have been 'heterosexually normal'. Other than conventional heterosexual, sexualities have to be explicitly revealed, and if one has found this difficult throughout one's younger years, in older age it is more difficult, especially within institutional care. If sexuality has become the prime medium through which people 'define their personalities ... establish their identities ... become conscious of themselves' (Foucault and Sennett, 1981: 22), for many elderly individuals the last vestiges of personality and identity are obliterated by societal and institutional silence over, and disinterest in, their sexualities.

Important elements in all social relationships are sexual relationships and interactions, whether sexual is defined in the broader aspects or in the more specific terms of sexual acts, orientations and relationships. For example 'attractive' physical appearance, in terms of hair and clothes, is considered a vital aspect of remaining a gendered and sexual individual, especially for women; there is rarely if ever any reference to older people (Hubbard *et al.*, 2004; Roach, 2004). Some older people do internalize the stereotype of the 'asexual older person' and are reluctant to discuss anything sexually related. This also appears to be compounded by societal perceptions that sex is not important for older people and may cause offence if discussed (Gott and Hinchliff, 2003). This will not be the case for all. One older person recently discussed in the *British Medical Journal* was actively seeking to meet his sexual needs.

A male resident in an older adult residential home was found to be paying a visitor for sex. What Barrett (2004) explores are the implications of the male resident procuring the services of a prostitute to meet his sexual needs while in a care environment. Staff preferred that the man be prescribed a drug to lower his libido, which Barrett describes feeling astonished at, and he therefore advocated on behalf of the gentleman. The debate rumbled on regarding whether he should have to spend his *own* money on such services. There was a marked improvement to his behaviour following sex and agreement from his family that the need existed for him. Unfortunately the debate was not resolved before the gentleman died. Surely we can make better sense of sexuality and have a 'grown-up' debate to resolve such issues for future individuals. As Barrett (2004) suggests, 'these circumstances will recur elsewhere', regardless of gender or sexuality.

Sexuality: experience and expression

How sexuality contributes to mental distress

Adequate sexual expression is essential to many human relationships and is an important aspect of life for most people (Higgins, Barker and Bageley, 2005). The whole subject is rarely understood and often cloaked in mystery and taboo or shrouded in idealized romance and fairytale. This is not confined to the institution but also occurs in society. The effects of sexuality and its expression can cause emotional difficulties and lead to further mental distress.

Early sociological accounts of sexuality asserted their terms of engagement to sceptics with some vigour: 'the sexual may be precisely that realm wherein the superordinate position of the socio-cultural order over the biological level is *most* complete' (Gagnon and Simon, 1973); 'sexuality is subject to socio-cultural moulding to a degree surpassed by few other forms of human behaviour' (1973); and pre-empted Foucault's later broad interpretation of the sexual within modernity's regime of 'bio-power' by claiming that 'nothing is sexual but naming it makes it so. Sexuality is a social construction learnt with others... The world is phenomenologically constructed and the interactionist unit of analysis is the ways in which sexual meanings are constructed, modified, negotiated, negated and constrained in conjoint action with others' (see Plummer, 1975: 29). The social construction of sexuality thus becomes inextricably tied to the social construction of mental ill-health: low self-esteem, concealment of personal issues of 'sexual' concern and inadequacy, drug and alcohol abuse, self-loathing and harm, depression, stress, anxiety, difficulty with intimacy, neuroses, even suicide.

The notion of lovesickness

It is argued by Langford that ideologies of romance have led women to believe that happiness is to be found through surrender to an idealized other, thus blinding them to the fact that heterosexual love relationships are both oppressive in themselves and play a crucial role in the maintenance of patriarchal society (Langford, 1997: 52).

Langford's research exposes a range of symptoms of physical and mental ill-health arising from 'love relationships', all suggestive of acute distress, including digestive upsets, weight loss, disruption of menstruation, chronic insomnia, depression, anxiety and eating disorders. Her respondents explained their ill health as being induced by what they perceived to be the emotional detachment of their male partners. They recognized these gendered disparities in the scripting of love and emotion as normal and natural and, as such, insuperable. To reiterate, they subscribed to the ideologies of innate male 'sex needs' and female 'innate attractiveness'. Men have sex; women have emotional attachments and relationships (McIntosh, 1978), ideologies which at the interpersonal level enable, it is argued, the use of emotional distancing by the male to exercise power and control over the female partner. The latter is forced into 'constriction of the self' (Symonds, 1974: 288): 'self-silencing' (losing sight of sense of self and feelings) and 'self-objectification' (learning to see herself as she imagines her partner sees her, and largely to her own detriment).

For instance one respondent, Jane, recounts:

> I went from, at one time, going very overweight from bingeing for comfort because I wasn't getting what I wanted out of the relationship, just eating, comfort eating, taking food to bed with me when he didn't realise – to going to the other extreme of making myself ill to ... diet drastically to try and be what he wanted me to be ... I developed stomach problems, and was nervous all the time.
> (Langford, 1997: 53)

The general complaint from the women in Langford's study was of their male partner's 'coldness' towards them. Natural conventional gender and sexual differences and their idealized but, in practice, failed resolutions through love, would appear to make mental ill-health an, albeit periodically, ubiquitous consequence of normal heterosexuality for women at least. Soaring divorce rates and an ever-increasing army of experts discoursing on the topic 'how to have a good relationship' suggest that, despite our aspirations, few are actually engaged in the emotionally satisfying, sexually fulfilling, compassionate relationship of the romantic ideal (Langford, 1997: 55).

Homophobia

By the end of the nineteenth century sexuality and mental health became formally conjoined in medical and legal discourse and practice, a conjunction further elaborated during the last third of the twentieth century with the extensive commodification of all aspects of sexuality, including many of those formerly labelled 'perverse', and 'mental health' in the leisure and 'life-style' consumption led economies of the first world. The nineteenth century had medicine and psychiatry effectively competing with religion and the law for jurisdiction over sexuality. As a consequence, discourse about homosexuality expanded from the realms of sin and crime to include that of pathology. This historical shift was generally considered progressive because a sick person was less blameful than a sinner or a criminal (Duberman, Vicinus and Chauncey, 1989). In 1952 the American Psychiatric Association included homosexuality as a sociopathic personality disorder in the first *Diagnostic and Statistical Manual of Psychiatric Disorders* and did not remove it until 1973.

Both male and female homosexuality have been fully medicalized since the late nineteenth century, medicalized as genetically, physiologically and psychologically abnormal conditions categorically set apart from the heterosexual majority. Historical studies tell us that prior to this discursive onslaught, homosexuality was recognized as behaviour which anyone was capable of indulging in, rather than a pathological condition defining a person's whole being (see Duberman *et al.*, 1989). Since the Labouchère Amendment to the Criminal Law Amendment Act (1885), male homosexual acts were outlawed as 'gross misdemeanours', until the limited Wolfenden Report (1957) inspired reforms almost a century later. But overall this Amendment, and subsequent legal measures, were informed by a medicalization of the homosexual (male) as a social threat, based on medical accounts of individual biological (physiological, genetic, chromosomal) but especially psychological pathologies.

Out of this threat emerges the context of homophobia, which is manifest as physical and verbal abuse, bullying, harassment and intimidation; rejection, exclusion, invalidation, marginalization, denial, making invisible, silencing; negative stereotyping, pathologization (seeing homosexuality as an illness or abnormality; believing that the problems that gay people experience are a result of their sexuality itself, rather than other people's treatment of them); teasing, joking, ridiculing, patronizing; discrimination, treating as second-class citizens; treating as sinful, immoral, predatory (devious and sly), dangerous to children (PACE, 2006: 1).

Unsurprisingly therefore, and despite the wide media attention focused on what is interpreted as evidence of greater social inclusion, the great majority of self-identified 'homosexuals', 'lesbians' and 'bisexuals' are not 'out' in significant areas of their lives. The mental health consequences are invariably therefore exacerbated by being tied to strategies of 'concealment' in a seemingly more tolerant but still hostile world. In such a context homophobia becomes just one more focus of stress inducing oppression, but seeking to politically counter it through adoption of its power-laden terminology is a grave mistake. While homophobia clearly signifies hostility to homosexuality and all things homosexual, on the grounds that heterosexuality is believed to be the only normal, valid and moral basis for sexual acts, identities, relationships and lifestyles, it is still a 'phobia', and thereby locked into an analytical paradigm of individual psychological shortcomings, rather than the result of the complex and duplicitous manoeuvrings of 'moral' states and amoral markets. Homophobia remains ensconced in an unchallenged dominant psychoanalytic paradigm, which confirms the 'otherness' of those who are its targets.

A study by Warner *et al.* (2004a) puts this into perspective, finding that gay men and lesbians living in England and Wales are at moderately increased risk of mental disorder and deliberate self-harm compared with heterosexual men and women. Some of the statistics identified that 42 per cent of gay men, 43 per cent of lesbians and 49 per cent of bisexual men and women had mental health problems. They concluded that these high levels of mental problems could be linked to discrimination due to sexuality, such as homophobia. Anxiety and depression, alongside considered and attempted suicide, are much higher in this population within the USA and UK (King and McKeown, 2003).

The impact of sexual expression in mental health care

Historically, sexual expression through masturbation has been thought to be the primary cause of many mental disorders. It has also been traditionally condemned by the Judeo-Christian religions, associating the loss of sperm for men with weakening of the body and spirit (Cort, Attenborough and Watson, 2001). However, masturbation, displays of affection, homosexuality, exhibitionism and intercourse are just some forms of sexual expression. So within mental health care common sense and clinical judgement should remain sensitive to the sexual needs of service users being able to express themselves and meet their needs (McCann, 2000).

There is a lack of published literature regarding sexual and relationship need and serious mental illness (McCann, 2003). Sexual need and expression in people with psychosis is not being addressed (McCann, 2000). When there actually is some discussion or realistic attempt at understanding, Deegan (1999) reminds us of the medical scrutiny of sexuality, with that which is private being under the lens for clinical and academic debate. Sexuality thus becomes the cause or symptom of psychopathology.

There is also a myth that people with mental illness have a lower sex drive. Buckley *et al.* (1999) suggest that 'decreased incidence is possibly due to low reporting and institutional segregation as opposed to an aspect of the illness'. Sexual activity among people with mental health problems is similar to that of the general population (Higgins *et al.*, 2005). People require privacy to express themselves and this may prove difficult under the gaze of staff. However, consideration is warranted for possible vulnerability to sexual exploitation (Higgins, Barker and Bageley, 2006).

Sexuality influenced by interaction

The impact of mental illness and mental health care on sexuality

The effects of the institution on sexual behaviour have received far less attention than the ways psychotropic medications impact sexual functioning and sex drive. Actually staying in a mental institution will take its toll on one's 'love life' (clinically defined as sexual interaction or activity). Room checks interfere with privacy when dressing, examining oneself or performing a sexual act, especially when staff do not knock or the room is shared by another person. This, as Deegan highlights, 'interferes with an adult's sexual activity, from self-masturbation to sexual intimacy with a partner' (Deegan, 1999). The situation requires careful consideration to balance staff responsibility versus service user autonomy.

Protecting and safeguarding persons with impaired decisional capacity are among the critical functions of a psychiatric hospital (Ford *et al.*, 2003; McCann, 2003). It may be both reasonable and prudent to prevent all sexual relationships between patients, as issues include transmission of sexually transmitted diseases, reproductive concerns and the legal implications of non-consensual activity (Ford *et al.*, 2003). All are no less of a concern for the general public, but sex is not banned or illegal. Personal liberty, sexual rights and freedom to consent should be the standard and the subject of sexuality afforded the mature acknowledgement it deserves. Prevention will serve no purpose. As Trudel and Desjardins (1994) state, 'problems associated with the expression of sexuality of patients in a psychiatric setting should be viewed through the principle of normalisation'. Another determining factor is through staff attitude. Most of the time staff are left with limited guidance and potential confusion in the event that a 'sexual incident' occurs (Ford *et al.*, 2003). In the care-home and nursing-home context, all residents will have elaborate sexual biographies, with potentially many 'sexual stories' (Plummer, 2003) to tell, but these stories are silenced (see Evans, 1999).

Care-settings studies show a marked lack of social interaction and activity between those in care with others in care and with their carers (see, e.g., Perrin, 1997; Roach, 2004). Indeed, institutionalization leads to 'iatrogenic loneliness' (Miles and Parker, 1999). However, the development and maintenance of social relationships in older age, particularly where it occurs, has been shown to significantly contribute to a person's health and related quality of life, life satisfaction and emotional, subjective and psychological well-being (see Kaplan, 1996; Hubbard *et al.*, 2003). These relationships have been chronicled as complex and diverse, with the great majority of studies of the elderly in care concentrating on issues relating to a secure sense of individual identity (Powers, 1996; Williams and Roberts, 1995), ignoring or avoiding aspects of sexual identity, orientation and experience.

In addition there is a dearth of information on sexuality in institutional care settings for older people, especially concerning residents with any degree of dementia (see Post, 2000; Series and Degano, 2005). In a general sense, care workers, relatives and residents themselves define the elderly as non-sexual, without sexual interests, identities, needs, capabilities or pasts, and if sexual needs and interests are shown in any explicit form, care workers seek to repress them (Brown, 1989; Glass, Mustan and Carter, 1986; Roach, 2004). More recently the importance of sexuality for older people has begun to be recognized (Holmes, Reingold and Teresi, 1997), and recommendations for care staff developed (Archibald, 2001; Sherman, 1999). There is evidence that for some residents, sexuality remains an important aspect of social identity (Nay, 1992) and, indeed, that some are engaged in sexual activity (Mulligan and Palguta, 1991; Roach, 2004).

Much of the evidence, however, centres on appearance, behaviours interpreted as flirtation, inevitably the use of much humour and innuendo and perhaps the need for physical touch, but where such behaviours tend towards the more explicit, the response from most care-home workers and residents is to label such tendencies disgusting or perverted. Under these circumstances it is unsurprising that the sexual interests, identities and needs, and perhaps most importantly the rich biographies, of 'homosexuals', 'lesbians', 'bisexuals' and 'transvestites' are simply not recognized or heard. Nor is there reference to issues of 'sexual harassment' or indeed the needs of those wishing to consummate sexual relations. Not only are the elderly generally regarded as non-sexual (Roach, 2004), but they are also, as a result, regarded as non-'sexual citizens'.

In the institutional services of mental health care, sexuality is a hidden aspect. It does not seem to be taken seriously or even seen as necessary (even though it is listed as a basic human need in such models as Maslow's hierarchy), and is generally considered perverted or deviant when the subject arises within the service. Add to this the possibility that the sexuality of the service user may be other than heterosexual and a purposeful dismissal may ensue. However, it is a basic human right.

Mossman *et al.* (1997) also asked the question, 'should psychiatric inpatients be allowed to engage in sexual activities?' This issue has received very little attention and there is a general assumption that people with schizophrenia 'don't have sex' (McCann, 2000). Buckley and Hyde (1997) surveyed staff at 86 state facilities across the USA for people suffering from mental illness. They found that 88 per cent of the 57 respondents considered sexual behaviour to be a clinical problem and most had policies addressing concerns and some form of psycho-educational programme. Warner *et al.* (2004b) recognize that 'sexual activity between service users raises special difficulties regarding consent…there is conflict between the individual's right to sexual expression and the need to protect vulnerable people'. However, Cort *et al.* (2001) found that support for service users and any sexual health education was marginalized because of other statutory commitments.

With regard to human sexuality and mental health it is imperative that clinicians' help clients keep the valued social roles they already have – as lover, spouse, partner, parent, grandparent. Although some clinicians view these roles as stressors, they are also a powerful motivating force for recovery (Deegan, 1999). The stigma of having a diagnosis such as schizophrenia compounded by misconceptions of society can lead to ostracism and alienation and may affect the formation and maintenance of intimate relationships (McCann, 2003). By developing and delivering sexual health-education programmes to staff and service user alike, people with mental health problems will be helped to develop intimacy skills and sexually healthy relationships and to overcome some of the social isolation and loneliness that they experience (McCann, 2004). Maturity, compassion, understanding and a reasonable, dignified approach to the subject of sexuality and mental health is warranted, whether sexual issues are a consequence of mental ill-health or visa versa.

However, when considering addressing the issue of sexuality in health, it appears clinicians are poor. In a recent survey of nurses conducted by Magnan and Reynolds (2006), they discovered that the number one barrier to nurses addressing service-user concerns over sexuality was the nurses' perception that service users 'do not expect nurses to address the sexuality concerns'. They also found that nurses lack confidence and do not feel comfortable addressing sexuality (Magnan and Reynolds, 2006). Indeed, many nurses do believe that sexuality assessment, evaluation and counselling is part of their professional role, but have not integrated this awareness into their care provision (Reynolds and Magnan, 2005).

It should also not be assumed that nurses have the necessary knowledge and skills to facilitate sexual health-education programmes (Higgins, Barker and Bageley, 2006). Indeed, before nurses can assist others with sex and relationship needs, they must examine their own attitudes, values, fears and beliefs. There should be much more of a drive to facilitate and promote communication about sexuality (McCann, 2003). This could begin in training and pre-registration education. There may also be scope to introduce the concept of acknowledging sexuality and its importance through interprofessional education.

Policy making

Policies to aid staff interpretation and understanding are scarce (Buckley and Robben, 2000). One of the few hospitals identifying need for a balanced policy is Riverview Hospital in British Columbia, Canada which created a task force to address the issue of sexual expression, activity and needs in its hospital (Welch and Clements, 1996). It reviewed the available literature, interviewed service users and conducted a formal survey of sexual behaviour and needs. Four general findings were revealed from the literature, including:

1. Many psychiatric service users hospitalized with chronic mental disorders are sexually active.
2. Addressing sexual needs often results in a sex education group.
3. Hospital staff have many concerns regarding service user sexuality, such as behaviour, expression, privacy, disease and moral issues.
4. The need for a formal policy has been recognised for some time, but remains virtually non-existent.

Welch and Clements (1996)

Service user interviews and a formal survey of sexual behaviour found that 39 per cent had no concerns with their sex life, 21 per cent did not reply and 40 per cent listed concerns ranging from lack of privacy, having no partner, no time with their partner, contraception, side effects of medication and unwanted advances from the opposite sex. The nurses returned questionnaires for all patients and perceived 15 per cent to have a problem with sexual behaviour. Problems ranged from exhibitionism, inappropriate propositions, sex in public, sexual assault, sexual abuse of oneself, innuendo and not practising safe sex. A new policy on patient sexuality was introduced at Riverview Hospital that consisted of several sections (see Appendix 1). Of the changes that took place, the bravest and yet most responsible was the introduction of a private suite for service users to utilise with consenting partners. The one stipulation was completion of their sex education programme before being able to access the suite. This demonstrated maturity and responsibility on the part of the hospital and service user.

The impact of psychotropic medication

Sexual dysfunction is a common side effect of psychotropic medication and is underestimated in the management of service users on long-term antipsychotic treatment (Smith and Gillam, 2005). Sexual dysfunction also occurs for almost half those taking antipsychotic medication. If asked directly about side effects, service users report high levels of sexual dysfunction. A recent survey by Rethink (2002) highlights that people treated for schizophrenia identify sexual dysfunction as the least tolerable side effect of antipsychotic medications. 'They [mental health professionals] want us to commit sexual suicide' (one service user's sentiments as reported in Deegan, 1999). The experience of iatrogenic sexual dysfunction is often minimized or ignored (Higgins, Barker and Bageley, 2005), with many service users given antipsychotic medications and not informed about the possible sexual dysfunction related to medication use (Deegan, 1999; Higgins *et al.*, 2005). Information, education, treatment choice and increased collaboration are necessary in order to take the impact of sexual dysfunction seriously and responsibly.

Moving forward

Policy can assist people with mental illness in the institutional cloak that denies sexuality. A more adult and responsible approach is warranted from the services. This will be further enhanced if the staff receive appropriate training to help understand and deal with the emergence of sexual need (King and McKeown, 2003), again, from an adult and responsible platform. If this leads to acceptance then it will be worth the effort. Even if the only acceptance is professional adherence to a considered and balanced policy that overrides personal opinion, it will be worth it.

Several of the most recent studies propose that staff education and training should be provided to highlight the importance of sexuality and sexual expression and to identify their own prejudice on the subject of older people, people with mental illness and sex (Gott and Hinchliff, 2003; Holmes *et al.*, 1997; Roach, 2004). Few hospitals actually specify that staff should receive specific training (Buckley and Robben, 2000). Higgins *et al.* (2006) explored the literature around the provision of sexual health-education for people with mental health problems. They found that a variety of programmes are provided. Most focus on HIV and other sexually transmitted diseases, along with negotiating safe sex, and skill development in condom use. They concluded that it is important to consider integrating such education with service provision. Some concerns are raised around fears that education may encourage sexual disinhibition, promiscuity and preoccupation. There is no evidence for this.

For one example of the benefits of education, Sladyk (1990) developed a 45-minute sexual health-education programme entitled 'AIDS Education and Safe Sex' for women in a locked psychiatric unit in the USA. At each session she described taking considerable time discussing the myths surrounding AIDS and techniques of safe sex. Following a post-test, Sladyk established that the women had increased their knowledge. Also, the programme had a record number of attendees. Unfortunately such programmes are rarely offered routinely. This also occurs for therapeutic input with sexual difficulties, such as psychosexual interventions, which is not usually offered to people with mental illness. In light of the emergence of a younger service user group, where expectations are quite different around sex and relationship issues; new challenges are being posed for mental health professionals (McCann, 2003).

Policy can inform the staff and service user as to the appropriate, responsible way forward in dealing with sexual matters. With the example of Riverview Hospital, British Columbia, discussed earlier, the provision of an actual private suite for service users to utilise with a consenting adult partner provides a safe place for intimacy and privacy (point 2 of the policy in Appendix 1). This concept is virtually unknown anywhere in the world to date and is quite possibly the only way forward for mental health care.

Conclusion

Many cultural taboos remain in addressing sexuality with vulnerable people (McCann, 2003). The issue of human sexuality presents mental health professionals with some of the most difficult ethical, moral and legal problems (McCann, 2000). Mental health care and the professionals working in its service provision will need to give consideration to the concept of sexuality, matched with the age of the service user and how it influences their care.

There are dark forces at work that impact on some people being able to express their sexuality or feel comfortable in showing their sexual orientation. The influence on a person's mental health is immense. Equally, the impact of mental health care on sexuality is immense too. Not only are there distress, symptoms, diagnoses and depleted confidence to contend with, but the treatment and care aspect of mental health impact even further to deny a side of human nature that should be considered central to core identity. Hopefully, the situation and approach will improve to embrace a mature and responsible future outlook for all concerned.

Appendix I

Policy on Sexual Rights at Riverview Hospital, British Columbia, Canada

1. The rights of patients within the hospital, including staff acceptance, hospital responsibility and balancing the rights of the patient with the responsibility of the hospital.

2. The environment and provision of privacy, to include a private suite for sexual intimacy.

3. A treatment protocol was included with respect to sexual issues.

4. An exclusive protocol for masturbation was deemed necessary as it was the most prevalent sexual activity.

5. Access to the private suites for intimacy and privacy required defining and cited a number of conditions, so as to protect the client and service.

6. This aspect incorporates the reality that the policy is untested and so is a 'get out clause' for professionals to over-ride any aspect.

7. The seventh section is provision for a review one year from introduction. The policy received full support from all management levels.

(Welch and Clements, 1996)

EDITORS' QUESTIONS

Issues of difference

▓ What are the gender issues with regard to sexual orientation?

▓ Can the sexual expression of a service user ever be acceptable?

▓ What cultural differences are there with regard to sexuality?

Relevance to practice

▓ Are you and your colleagues able and comfortable to address sexual needs with service users?

▓ In what way is a person's sexual orientation considered?

▓ Which professional discipline is best placed to deal with the sexual needs of a service user?

Investigate

▓ How is staff homophobia addressed in clinical training and education?

▓ How can sexuality be enabled to be expressed during a long period of hospital admission?

▓ To what degree does sexual dysfunction occur for people taking psychotropic medications?

Suggested further reading

Buckley, P. (ed.) (1999) *Sexuality and Serious Mental Illness*. Amsterdam: Harwood Academic.
Foucault, M. (1981) *The History of Sexuality, Volume One: An Introduction*. Harmondsworth: Penguin.

References

Archibald, C. (2001) Resident sexual expression and the key worker relationship: and unspoken stress in residential care work', *Practice*, **13**(1): 5–12.

Barrett, J. (2004) Personal services or dangerous liaisons: should we help patients hire prostitutes? *British Medical Journal*, **329**: 985.

Brown, L. (1989) Is there sexual freedom for our aging population in long-term care institutions? *Journal of Gerontological Social Work*, **13**: 75–93.

Buckley, P.F. and Hyde, J.L. (1997) State hospitals' responses to the sexual behaviour of psychiatric inpatients. *Psychiatric Services*, **48**(3): 398–9.

Buckley, P.F., Robben, T., Friedman, L., and Hyde, J. (1999) Sexual behaviour in people with serious mental illness: patterns and clinical correlates. In: P. Buckley, *Sexuality and Serious Mental Illness*. Amsterdam: Harwood Academic.

Buckley, P.F. and Robben, T. (2000) A content analysis of state hospital policies on sex between inpatients. *Psychiatric Services*, **51**(2): 243–5.

Cort, E.M., Attenborough, J., and Watson, J.P. (2001) An initial exploration of community mental health nurses' attitudes to and experience of sexuality-related issues in their work with people experiencing mental health problems. *Journal of Psychiatric and Mental Health Nursing*, **8**: 489–99.

Deegan, P.E. (1999) Human sexuality and mental illness: Consumer viewpoints and recovery principles. In P. Buckley (ed.) *Sexuality and Serious Mental Illness*. Amsterdam: Harwood Academic, pp. 21–33.

Duberman, M.B., Vicinus, M. and Chauncey, G. (1989) *Hidden from History: Reclaiming the Gay and Lesbian Past*. New York: Dutton Adult.

Evans, D.T. (1999) The eighth age of man: sociological reflections on Alzheimer's Disease. In: M.V. Morrissey and A Coakley (eds) *Alzheimer's Disease: Beyond the Medical Model*. Trowbridge: Quay Books, pp. 27–42.

Ford, E., Rosenberg, M., Holsten, M. and Boudreaux, T. (2003) Managing sexual behaviour on adult acute care inpatient psychiatric units. *Psychiatric Services*, **54**(3): 346–50.

Foucault, M. and Sennett, R. (1981) Sexuality and solitude. *Humanities in Review*, **1**(3): 21.

Gagnon, J.H. (1967) Sexuality and sexual learning in the child. In J.H. Gagnon and W.S. Simon (eds) *Sexual Deviance*. London: Harper & Row.

Gagnon, J.H. and Simon, W.S. (1973) *Sexual Conduct: The Social Sources of Human Sexuality*. Chicago: Aldine.

Glass, J., Mustan, R., and Carter, L. (1986) Knowledge and attitudes of health-care providers towards sexuality in the institutionalized elderly. *Educational Gerontology*, **12**: 465–75.

Gott, M. and Hinchliff, S. (2003) Barriers to seeking treatment for sexual problems in primary care: a qualitative study with older people. *Family Practice*, **20**: 690–5.

Greer, G. (1984) *Sex and Destiny: The Politics of Human Fertility*. London: Secker & Warburg.

Heath, S. (1982) *The Sexual Fix*. London: Macmillan.

Higgins, A., Barker, P., and Bageley, C.M. (2005) Neuroleptic medication and sexuality: the forgotten aspect of education and care. *Journal of Psychiatric and Mental Health Nursing*, **12**: 439–46.

Higgins, A., Barker, P., and Bageley, C.M. (2006) Sexual health education for people with mental health problems: what can we learn from the literature? *Journal of Psychiatric and Mental Health Nursing*, **13**: 687–97.

Holmes D., Reingold, J., and Teresi, J. (1997) Sexual expression and dementia. *International Journal of Geriatric Psychiatry*, **12**(7): 695–701.

Hubbard, G., Cook, A., Tester, S., and Downs, M. (eds) (2003) *Sexual Expression in Institutional Care Settings for Older People*, Stirling: University of Stirling Department of Film and Media Studies (interactive CD).

Kaplan L. (1996) Sexual and institutional issues when one spouse resides in the community and the other lives in a nursing home, *Sexuality and Disability*, **14**(4), 281–94.

King, M. and McKeown, E. (2003) *Mental Health and Social Well-Being of Gay Men, Lesbians and Bisexuals in England and Wales*. MIND.

Langford, W. (1997) 'You make me sick': Women, health and romantic love. *Journal of Contemporary Health*, **5**: 52–5.

Lees, S. (1993) *Sugar and Spice*. London: Penguin.

Mac an Ghail, M. (1994) *The Making of Men*. Milton Keynes: Open University Press.

Magnan, M.A. and Reynolds, K.E. (2006) Barriers to addressing patient sexuality concerns across five areas of specialization, *Clinical Nurse Specialist*, **20**(6): 285–92.

McCann, E. (2000) The expression of sexuality in people with psychosis: breaking the taboos. *Journal of Advanced Nursing*, **32**(1): 132–8.

McCann, E. (2003) Exploring sexual relationship possibilities for people with psychosis: a review of the literature. *Journal of Psychiatric and Mental Health Nursing*, **10**: 640–9.

McCann, E. (2004) The sexual and relationship needs of people with psychosis living in the community. PhD Thesis, City University, London. Cited in A. Higgins, P. Barker, and C.M. Bageley (2006), Sexual health education for people with mental health problems: what can we learn from the literature? *Journal of Psychiatric and Mental Health Nursing*, **13**: 687–97.

McIntosh, M. (1978) Who needs prostitutes?: The ideology of male sex needs and female attractiveness. In C. Smart and B. Smart (eds.) *Women, Sexuality and Social Control*. London: Routledge & Kegan Paul.

Mental Health Foundation (2006) Latest news on gender, sexuality and mental health, schools should teach about loving sex, parents say. http://www.mentalhealth.org.uk/information/news/?q=0,23/05/2006,&EntryId=32000 [accessed 28/05/07].

Miles, S. and Parker, K. (1999) 'Sexuality in the nursing home: iatregenic loneliness. *Generations*, **Spring**: 36–43.

Mossman, D., Perlin, M.L. and Dorfman, D.A. (1997) Sex on the wards: Conundra for clinicians. *Journal of the American Academy of Psychiatry and the Law*, **25**(4): 441–60.

Mulligan, T. and Palguta, R. (1991) Sexual interest, activity and satisfaction among Male nursing home residents. *Archives of Sexual Behaviour*, **20**: 199–205.

Nay, R. (1992) Sexuality and aged women in nursing homes. *Geriatric Nursing*, **11**: 312–14.

PACE (2006) Good practice guidelines for the mental health services. http://www.pacehealth.org.uk/guidelines.html

Perrin, T. (1997) Occupational need in severe dementia: a descriptive study. *Journal of Advanced Nursing*, **25**: 934–41.

Plummer, K. (1975) *Sexual Stigma: An Interactionist Account*. London: Routledge & Kegan Paul.

Plummer, K. (2003) Intimate citizenship and the culture of sexual story telling. In J. Weeks., J. Holland, and S. Waites (eds) *Sexualities and Society*. Cambridge: Polity Press.

Post, S. (2000) Commentary on sexuality and intimacy in the nursing home. *Journal of Clinical Ethics*, **11**: 314–17.

Powers, B. (1996) Relationships among older women living in a nursing home. *Journal of Women and Aging*, **8**: 179–98.

Rethink (2002) *A Question of Choice*. http://www.mentalhealthshop.org/products/rethink_publications/question_of.html [accessed 08/06/07].

Reynolds, K.E. and Magnan, M.A. (2005) Nursing attitudes and beliefs toward human sexuality: collaborative research promoting evidence-based practice. *Clinical Nurse Specialist*, **19**(5): 255–9.

Roach, S.M. (2004) Sexual behaviour of nursing home residents: staff perceptions and responses. *Journal of Advanced Nursing*, **48**(4): 371–9.

Series, H. and Degano, P. (2005) Hypersexuality in dementia, *Advances in Psychiatric Treatment*, **11**: 424–31.

Sherman, B. (1999) *Sexuality, Intimacy and Aged Care*. London: Jessica Kingsley.

Sladyk, K. (1990) Teaching safe sex practices to psychiatric patients. *American Journal of Occupational Therapy*, **44**(3): 284–6.

Smith, S. and Gillam, T. (2005) Sexual dysfunction: the forgotten taboo. *Mental Health Nursing Journal*, 25(1): 6–9.

Symonds, A. (1974) Phobias after marriage: Women's declaration of dependence. In J.B. Miller (ed.) *Psychoanalysis and Women*. Penguin: Harmondsworth.

Trudel, G. and Desjardins, G. (1994) Sexuality in the psychiatric milieu. *Canadian Journal of Psychiatry*, 39(7): 421–8.

Warner, J., McKeown, E., Griffin, M., Johnson, K., Ramsay, A., Cort, C., and King, M. (2004a) Rates and predictors of mental illness in gay men, lesbians and bisexual men and women. *British Journal of Psychiatry*, 185: 479–85.

Warner, J., Pitts, N., Crawford, M.J., Serfaty, M., Prabhakaran, P. and Amin, R. (2004b) Sexual activity among patients in psychiatric hospital wards. *Journal of the Royal Society of Medicine*, 97(10): 477–9.

Welch, S.J. and Clements, G.W. (1996) Development of a policy on sexuality for hospitalized chronic psychiatric patients. *Canadian Journal of Psychiatry*, 41(5): 273–9.

WHO (World Health Organization), Gender and Reproductive Rights: http://www.who.int/reproductive-health/gender/sexual_health.html [accessed 25/08/07].

Williams, B. and Roberts, P. (1995) Friends in passing: social interaction at an adult day care centre. *International Journal of Aging and Human Development*, 41: 63–78.

Wolfenden Report (1957) *The Report of the Committee on Homosexual Offences and Prostitution*, Cmnd 247. London: HMSO.

Worldwide Ages of Consent, http://www.avert.org/aofconsent.htm [accessed 14/09/07].

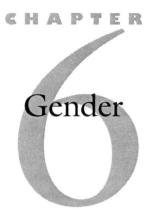

CHAPTER

6

Gender

Vicki Coppock

BRIEF CHAPTER OUTLINE

This chapter critically examines the way in which gender discrimination features in the lives of people in mental distress. Discussion will incorporate the social construction of gender through the patriarchal construct of masculinity and mainly femininity. This leads to a gender bias in mental health research towards women and their assumed greater vulnerability or proneness to mental disorder. It is thus argued that mental health knowledge is inaccurate in the absence of good critical research. Gendered patterns are then explored for prevalence, risk factors and help seeking. Following a brief look at changing gender roles in the twenty-first century, the chapter moves to highlight women's experience specifically in the mental health system. The conclusion focuses on mainstreaming gender and future visions that would see women (in particular) reporting improved service.

Introduction

In recent years there has been a growing expectation that the mental health system and professionals within it become more sensitive to the dynamics of discrimination and oppression in the lives of people in mental distress. The ways in which systematic forms of oppression and discrimination (class, race, ethnicity, age, sexuality and gender) may cause or exacerbate mental health problems has been articulated in government policy (DH, 1999, 2000, 2002a, 2003, 2005; NIMHE, 2003, 2004, Scottish Government, 2006), in professional education and training developments (GSCC, 2002; SCMH, 2001), in voluntary sector/service-user publications such as *Asylum*; *OpenMind* and *MadNation*, and in the wider academic literature (Barnes and Bowl, 2001; Rogers and Pilgrim, 2003; Sayce, 2000; Tew, 2005).

This chapter critically examines the way in which gender discrimination in particular features in the lives of people in mental distress and the implications of this for mental health practitioners. This includes a discussion of the social construction of gender; the patriarchal nature of mental health theory, research and practice; gendered patterns of mental distress; and women's experiences of the mental health system. Recent efforts to address gender inequality in mental health policy and professional practice in the UK are outlined and critically examined. The chapter addresses the fundamental question 'what needs to be done in order to achieve a gender-sensitive mental health system'?

According to the Beijing Platform for Action (1995, cited in DH, 2002a: 26), 'the term "gender" refers to the economic, social, political and cultural attributes and opportunities associated with being male and female'. 'Gender', therefore, describes *socially determined* characteristics of women and men whereas 'sex' is *biologically determined*. Gender is fundamental to identities, roles and relationships. It is not merely about differences between men and women but also about inequality.

'In most societies, men and women differ in the activities they undertake, in access and control of resources, and in participation in decision-making. In most societies women as a group have less access than men to resources, opportunities and decision-making' (ibid.: 26).

The term 'sexism' is used to describe inequality, discrimination and oppression on the grounds of gender. Sexism operates at the *personal* level of individual beliefs and actions, at the *cultural* level of values and norms and at the *structural* level of institutions (Thompson, 2001). At each level there exists an inherent bias against women that generates and sustains systematic disadvantage in all areas of women's lives. The term 'patriarchy' (literally 'law of the father') refers to the dominance of men both within the family and in society in general. Sexism reinforces and is reinforced by patriarchy. It is a system that meets men's needs at women's expense. More specifically in the context of this chapter, sexism and patriarchy create, maintain and exacerbate exposure to risk factors that endanger women's mental health. This implies that practitioners need to radically rethink the male-dominated basis of mental health theory, research, policy and practice.

'We are not able as professionals to intervene appropriately or justly in people's lives unless we perceive the ways in which women are disadvantaged by an unequal dispersal of power, and in which both men and women are constrained by over-rigid and falsely dichotomised role and relationship expectations' (Mullender, 1997).

Patriarchal processes in mental health theory, research and practice

All assessments of mental health depend on theories of human behaviour – what is believed to constitute the normal and how this can be distinguished from the pathological. Theories about the causes of mental distress vary between, and, to some extent, within, the various disciplines concerned with the field of mental health, though most conform to what is termed the *medical model*. The medical model emerged from the mid-nineteenth century onwards, shifting earlier moral or religious frameworks of explanation for mental distress towards an illness framework that embraces organic, social and psychological explanations. The modern-day language and practice of mental health mimics that of the medical sciences with the belief that mental health diagnosis simply involves the accurate naming of an objective disease process (Bracken and Thomas, 2000). However, critical theorists and researchers have revealed how diagnosis depends largely on the subjective judgement of one individual – a psychiatrist – who is often male, white and middle-class (Loring and Powell, 1988; see also chapter 1).

It is of particular significance to this chapter that many traditional theories of mental health and illness reflect androcentric bias, where men's experiences are taken as the norm and/or their symptoms and patterns of distress are used to inform models of explanation. Various researchers and writers, particularly from within feminism, support the assertion that the mental health system is imbued with sexist ideology and, as a result, discriminates against women in mental distress (Glick *et al.*, 2000; Penfold and Walker, 1984; Prior, 1999; Russell, 1995; Ussher, 1991). They demonstrate how the construction of disease categories, biases in psychiatric assessment and the socialization of gendered psychologies all contribute to an understanding of gender and mental health. While there are a number of different positions in feminist theorizing on women's mental health, there is a common concern with the significance of patriarchy in mental health theory, research and practice.

Critical perspectives: social construction or social causation?

Some theorists have argued that a mental health diagnosis is not an illness as such but a label attached to women who step outside the boundaries of acceptable femininity (Chesler, 1972; Penfold and Walker, 1984; Ussher, 1991). They suggest that notions of acceptable and unacceptable feminine behaviour have helped to shape expectations and understandings of women's mental distress for those who use mental health services and for those who provide such services. These writers point to the significance of patriarchal power structures in defining mental distress and how this contributes to the overrepresentation of women as 'mad'. Chesler's influential study *Women and Madness* (1972) reveals how gender is embedded in the very construction of concepts of madness and mental illness. She argues that the simple act of deviating from the roles expected of men and women in a patriarchal society can lead to definitions of mental disorder. However, for women there is a double bind since in patriarchal societies masculinity is privileged and femininity devalued. Therefore women who both conform to or depart from their sex-role stereotype are liable to attract diagnoses of mental disorder. This argument is supported by a well-known study by Broverman *et al.* (1970). These researchers examined clinicians' understandings of mental health and illness, revealing the operation of gender-based stereotypes. Psychological ill-health was consistently associated with the feminine stereotype.

Other studies have confirmed that mental health professionals are more likely to equate feminine characteristics with mental ill-health (Corob, 1987; Penfold and Walker, 1984; Sheppard, 1991; WHO, 2001). For these researchers the *social construction* of women as essentially mentally unstable is one manifestation of the patriarchal control of women. The labelling process functions to maintain women's position as outsiders, dismiss women's anger as illness and explain women's unhappiness as some internal flaw, obscuring the need to question the social structures of patriarchy. Moreover, this process operates over time with the labels changing according to prevailing discourses. So, for example, Showalter (1987) argues that Victorian discourses around femininity produced constructions of women's deviancy that were labelled as hysteria or neurasthenia, while in the twentieth century these were replaced by labels such as anxiety, depression and anorexia nervosa.

Historically, madness has been associated with femininity and the female body. Indeed, the connection of a woman's mental distress with her biology is one of the most powerful discourses bearing down on women (Ehrenreich and English, 1979; Foucault, 1967; Showalter, 1987). Ordinary functions of the female life cycle such as menstruation, pregnancy and the menopause have been pathologized and psychiatrized. Biological explanations of women's mental distress continue to dominate mental health theory and practice today, even though 'recent research suggests that the impact of biological and reproductive factors on women's mental health is strongly mediated and, in many cases disappears, when psychosocial factors are taken into account' (WHO, 2001: 8). Feminist writers would argue that the overemphasis on biologically based theories of gender differences in mental health reflects sexist assumptions and ideologies more than scientific fact.

Another theoretical perspective on gender and mental distress acknowledges the reality of women's mental distress but explains it as a consequence of living in an oppressive patriarchal society. This is referred to as the *social causation* model. It emphasizes the significance of the social circumstances of women's everyday lives, including gendered sources of stress and their impact on women (Stoppard, 1997). In patriarchal society women are socially disadvantaged by the roles they are expected to perform, and they have restricted access to the resources that promote good mental health (money and paid work). The particular stresses women are exposed to – economic dependence, familial caring responsibilities, social isolation, physical and sexual abuse – have all been identified as significant factors making them vulnerable to mental distress (WHO, 2000). This will be discussed in more detail later in the chapter.

Feminist approaches make an important contribution to our understanding of the way in which gender inequality features in the lives of women mental health service users. They offer practitioners a valuable critique of the traditional knowledge base for professional practice (i.e. the medical model) and its failure to get to grips with the roots and context of women's distress. They expose patriarchal processes in the conceptualization and treatment of mental distress. Nevertheless, women in mental distress live their lives within a complex range of determining contexts. Therefore to focus exclusively on the universal category of 'woman' is insufficient if practitioners are to fully appreciate the diversity of those experiences. Other dimensions of structured inequality that feature in women's lives – racism, poverty, ageism and homophobia – must all be acknowledged and responded to.

Similarly, it is important that a full understanding of men's, as well as women's, experiences of mental distress is developed since both are adversely affected by gender stereotyping and inequality in the mental health system. Patriarchal constructions of masculinity as well as femininity may contribute to experiences of mental distress for some men. Research by Warren (1983) reveals how men may find it difficult to recognize and seek help for depressive symptoms since depression is 'incompatible' with masculinity. Courtenay (2000) explains, 'the denial of depression is one of the means men use to demonstrate masculinities and to avoid assignment to a lower-status position relative to women and other men'. However, as White (2002: 275) argues, 'the "ideal man" is an abstract fiction that few men have the cultural or economic resources to attain in the course of their lives'. This is perhaps most forcefully indicated in the rising incidence of suicide among young men – a topic that will be returned to later in the chapter.

Gender bias in mental health research

It is clear from the above discussion that what is 'known' about men's and women's mental health has been significantly shaped by patriarchy, and this includes the process of knowledge creation itself. Traditional research has reflected the male domination of knowledge in terms of what is considered worthy of study, how research is managed and how results are presented. Historical and contemporary biases in mental health research have resulted in a distorted and incomplete understanding of the relationship between gender and mental health. Research into male mental disorder has been rare in comparison to the literature on women's mental health. This is because gender-blind theories of mental health have gone hand in hand with research that has assumed, and then sought evidence to prove, women's greater vulnerability or proneness to mental disorder (WHO, 2001).

When sex (a biological given) and gender (a social and cultural construct) are conflated this leads to systematic bias. For example, as discussed earlier, the relationship of women's reproductive functioning to their mental health has received intense scrutiny, yet the contribution that men's reproductive functioning might make to their mental health has been virtually ignored (WHO, 2001). This form of gender bias implies that men either have no reproductive functioning or are not psychologically affected by events and conditions related to reproduction such as infertility, miscarriage, stillbirth, prematurity or the transition to parenthood. It is inconceivable that men are not affected emotionally by many of the same events that influence women's emotional well-being. For example, more recent research has shown that men can also experience mental distress during pregnancy and following the birth of a child (Condon, Boyce and Corkindale, 2004; Soliday, McCluskey-Fawcett and O'Brien, 1999).

Similarly, the relatively late inclusion of violence against women into the mental health research agenda is another example of the way in which gender can influence the generation of a research problematic. Evidence on the relationship between gender-based, intimate violence and women's mental health has only been sought consistently over the last decade (WHO, 2000). Prior to this even social models of mental health neglected the significance of childhood sexual abuse or partner violence as potential vulnerability factors in the development of depression and other forms of mental distress.

As discussed earlier, gender intersects with other forms of structural inequality such as race, class, age and sexuality. Racism, poverty and isolation shape the lives, opportunities and experiences of women who use mental health services (Buck, 1997; Sheppard, 2002; Wilson, 2001). In the mainstream research literature (and thereby in professional practice) the specific experiences and needs of these women have been invisible. Likewise, although it is encouraging to see some research that reflects the complexities of experiences of mental distress for older women (Barnes, 1997), disabled women (Morris, 2004), lesbian women and gay men (King *et al.*, 2003; McFarlane, 1998), such research has proved slow to penetrate the mainstream.

Together, these examples demonstrate that without the incorporation of good quality critical research about gender and mental health into mental health education and training, mental health practitioners' knowledge will be inaccurate and incomplete. Therefore all levels of scientific enquiry, from the formulation of research questions through to design, methodology and interpretation of results, need to explicitly articulate the contribution of gender. There is a compelling need to rectify the effect of gender bias in mental health research so that the evidence base serves to reliably inform practitioners' understanding of gender differences in mental health and, crucially, their practice.

Gendered patterns of mental distress

Although at a variety of levels the evidence base is highly contested, it is nonetheless clear that gender differences in mental health do exist. Socially constructed differences between men and women in terms of their roles and responsibilities, status and power interact with biological differences between the sexes. This leads to differential experiences of mental distress, differential reporting of mental distress and differential responses to that distress from health and social care professionals and society as a whole.

According to the World Health Organization (WHO, 2002), gender is a critical determinant of mental health and mental illness in a global context. However, more is known about gender and mental health in industrialized countries than in the developing world. Studies in the general population suggest that the overall prevalence of mental distress is more or less the same for men and women (Kessler *et al.*, 1994). Nevertheless, significant gender differences do emerge in relation to specific disorders. For example women predominate in the rates of common mental disorders such as anxiety and depression, eating disorders and post-traumatic stress disorder, while men predominate in prevalence rates for drug and alcohol dependence and anti-social personality disorder (Gold, 1998; Mental Health Foundation, 2003a, 2003b; WHO, 2002). In contrast to the marked gender differences in the rates of common mental disorders, few gender differences in prevalence have emerged from studies on severe mental disorders, such as schizophrenia and bipolar disorder (Kessler *et al.*, 1994; Office for National Statistics, 2001). Gender differences also exist in the patterns of help-seeking for mental distress. Research reveals that women are more likely to seek early help and get treatment from their general practitioner while men, who find it difficult to express emotional distress, present later and are more likely to be referred (WHO, 2002).

The World Health Organization predicts that depression will be the second leading cause of global disability by 2020 and the leading cause of disability for women in developing nations (WHO, 2000). Depression occurs approximately twice as often in women as it does in men and is the most frequently encountered women's mental health problem (Bebbington, 1996). Studies from industrialized countries report how exposure to uncontrollable life events such as illness and death of children or husbands, imprisonment, job insecurity, dangerous neighbourhoods and hazardous workplaces puts women at greater risk of depression than men (WHO, 2000). Additionally, research reveals other gender-specific risk factors for common mental disorders, such as depression, that have a disproportionate impact on women. These include poverty, single parenthood, unremitting caring responsibilities and intimate partner violence and sexual abuse (DH, 2002a; WHO, 2000).

Studies have consistently reported the close association between mental ill-health and poverty (Sheppard, 2002). While access to paid work usually acts as a protective factor for positive mental health, when it is poorly paid, of low status or carried out in stressful or hazardous conditions, it is a risk factor for negative mental health. In a world where women are routinely disadvantaged by gender inequalities this means that they are at much greater risk of being adversely affected by poverty than their male counterparts (Wetzel, 2000). Women in general are poorer and experience greater deprivation; have less social and political power and have less access to health, education and employment than men (WHO, 2001). Social and demographic changes have contributed to a substantial increase in the numbers of households headed by women. Lone mothers and older women are particularly vulnerable to poverty and therefore are at greater risk of mental distress (Bebbington, Targosz and Lewis, 2002; Doyal, 2000).

The care of sick and disabled relatives falls disproportionately on women and the long-term impact of this has significant implications for their mental health (Henwood, 1998; Singleton *et al.*, 2002). Research suggests that older women who have primarily worked within the domestic sphere are more likely to experience depression than those employed outside the home (Milne and Williams, 2003).

Studies in the UK and the USA reveal that at least half of women using mental health services have experienced sexual or physical abuse as children and/or adults (Itzen, 2006; McCauley *et al.*, 1997; Mullen *et al.*, 1993). The World Health Organization (2000) has also highlighted the disproportionate effects of violence and abuse on women in an international context. Research has documented an extensive range of negative mental health consequences for women following all forms of violence – physical, sexual and emotional. Women who have experienced violence, whether in childhood or adult life, have increased rates of depression and anxiety, post-traumatic stress disorder, phobias, chemical dependency, substance misuse and suicidal thoughts and behaviour (WHO, 2000; 2001).

Overall there is extensive high-quality research evidence to suggest that women's mental health could be significantly improved by women gaining control over the determinants of their mental health (in particular, eliminating situations where they are devalued and discriminated against); reducing the exposure of women to those risk factors which compromise their mental health (especially violence and abuse); and involving women in decision-making in *all* aspects of their lives. Clearly this research evidence needs to directly inform developments in mental health policy and practice and, as will be demonstrated towards the end of this chapter, there are signs that some progress is being made in this direction.

Gender in the twenty-first century: changing roles?

Until relatively recently there was a deeply held assumption that women are more mentally unstable than men. Epidemiological data appeared to support that viewpoint, with women being overrepresented in almost all mental health statistics. However, a growing body of research indicates changing gender patterns in the reporting, diagnosis and treatment of mental disorder. Evidence points to the increased visibility of young men in measures of psychiatric morbidity with significant rises in the rates of suicidal and para-suicidal behaviours, depressive disorders and adolescent conduct disorders (McQueen and Henwood, 2002). Hospital admission rates have also begun to show slightly higher rates of men than women in recent times (Healthcare Commission, 2007). This has prompted researchers and writers from various disciplines to theorize the reasons behind the changing profile of men's mental health.

Some writers point to the dislocation of 'postmodern' cultural identities (Frosh, 1997) to explain how social, political and economic changes in late modern society appear to have disrupted men's psychological health. Connell (1995) emphasizes the changes in gender relations that have gone hand in hand with these broader changes (notably the rise of feminism and the challenge to patriarchal power) and how they have contributed to a 'crisis' of masculinity. Changes to established gender patterns, both in the workplace and in personal relationships, have unsettled the traditional western view of masculinity with its emphasis on rationality and lack of emotion. It is possible that young men have found it increasingly difficult to define themselves as adult men in contemporary society, finding it 'difficult to exist within or find alternatives to the traditional, fragmented category of masculinity' (McQueen and Henwood, 2002).

With the exception of China and parts of India, the rate of death by suicide is higher for men than women in almost all parts of the world (although suicide *attempts* remain more common among women than men) (WHO, 2002). It has been suggested that younger men have become particularly vulnerable in the context of increasing unemployment, occupational uncertainty, widespread substance misuse and family/relationship breakdown (Hawton, 1998). Available research paints a picture of young men who are disengaged from both society and mainstream services (Spurrell, Hatfield and Perry, 2003). In the UK this has prompted the development of a range of mental health policy initiatives targeting this group, such as the Department of Health (2002a) *National Suicide Prevention Strategy* and the Scottish Government (2002) *Choose Life*.

According to Prior and Hayes (2001: 399), it is unclear whether the reported statistical changes reflect a real increase in mental distress among men or rather 'the male-derived re-conceptualisation of mental disorder'. They report that the attention of mental health professionals has shifted away from definitions of mental disorder which focus almost exclusively on conditions associated with women (i.e. anxiety and depression) towards those primarily associated with men (i.e. substance dependence and anti-social personality disorder). This process may have contributed to men's increased susceptibility to institutionalization. Indeed, evidence suggests that greater numbers of men find themselves the focus of the mental health system when notions of risk and potential dangerousness are high on the political agenda (Prior and Hayes, 2001).

The changing profile of men's mental health clearly has important implications for the provision of gender-sensitive mental health services. Gender differences in the reporting of mental distress may be attributed to the dominant western stereotype of men as 'emotionally illiterate', but there are clearly ways in which men are *constrained* from articulating their distress. Service providers and mental health professionals need to have an awareness of the changing context of men's and women's lives and to become more attuned to the specific ways in which young men talk about and make sense of their emotional distress to ensure an accurate understanding of that distress. Just as with women's mental health, there is a need to move beyond the taken-for-granted constructions of mental health that have detracted from the quality of mental health services to both sexes.

Women's experiences of the mental health system

Although women make up two-thirds of all mental health service users, those who design and manage those services are primarily men. This poses the fundamental question of how it is possible for mental health services to be truly gender sensitive while such an imbalance exists. Can it be assumed that women's needs and interests will be met regardless? On closer scrutiny it appears not.

Differential responses from health and social care professionals to men and women in mental distress have been documented for some time (Williams *et al.*, 1993). Research reveals that, although largely well-intentioned, mental health professionals often locate problems within women and ignore or deny the sociopolitical factors that are the context, and frequently the source, of their distress. As discussed earlier, many have double standards of mental health that have negative consequences for women (Chesler, 1972; Ehrenreich and English, 1979; Roberts, 1985).

Traditionally, women are more likely than men to be treated for a mental health problem and to be admitted to hospital (Payne, 1998 cited in Lester and Glasby, 2006). Gender bias and stereotyping in the treatment of female patients and in the diagnosis of psychological disorders has been reported since the 1970s (WHO, 2001). Researchers have found that doctors are more likely to diagnose depression in women compared with men, even when they have similar scores on standardized measures of depression or present with identical symptoms (Callahan *et al.*, 1997; Stoppe, Sandholzer and Huppertz, 1999).

The dominance of medical discourse in women's lives as a whole has been mirrored in the response to women's mental health. Women report that medication is often the only option made available to them (Resisters, 2002; Scott and Williams, 2001). Women are 48 per cent more likely than men to be prescribed psychotropic drugs (Simoni-Wastila, 2000). Rogers and Pilgrim (2003: 85) describe 'the gendered effects of iatrogenic drug prescribing' and in particular how the cavalier prescribing of benzodiazepines resulted in 'widespread addiction and the oppression of women'. Moreover they argue that the extensive use of the newer anti-depressants such as Prozac still represent a gendered and predominantly medicalized response to the social and personal troubles that arise out of familial, social and economic conditions. Women (particularly older women) are also more likely to receive ECT, while men are more likely to be referred by their GP to specialist services (Payne, 1998 cited in Lester and Glasby, 2006). Women have traditionally been more likely than men to be both assessed for compulsory detention under mental health legislation and sectioned following assessment (Barnes, Bowl and Fisher, 1990). This clearly raises important issues regarding the civil liberties of female service users.

The majority of mental health care for women in the UK is located in generic, mixed-sex services. There are some dedicated women-only services, though most of these are provided by the voluntary sector and there is great variability across the country. There have been serious criticisms of mixed gender mental health care. Grave concerns have been expressed about women's safety in a variety of residential mental health settings, especially in relation to experiences of harassment, intimidation, coercion, violence and sexual abuse by other service users, visitors or staff (DH, 2002a; Wood and Copperman, 1996).

Although mental health service users frequently report that they want greater access to 'talking treatments', critical research reveals that these are potentially no less problematic for women unless they are informed by a woman-centred approach. Ussher (1991) notes the way in which many conventional therapies encourage women to look inwardly for the source of their distress rather than to the wider social structure. Perhaps more disturbing is the extensive evidence of women's experiences of sexual oppression by male therapists, ranging from patronizing comments to sexual harassment, assault and rape (Chesler, 1972; Rutter, 1995; Wood, 1993; Wood and Copperman, 1996).

Mainstreaming gender in mental health policy and legislation

It has rarely been the case that women have been asked what they want from the mental health care system. The exception has been those smaller-scale projects that are committed to listening to and empowering women in mental distress (see Barnes and Bowl, 2001; Good Practices in Mental Health, 1994). The campaigning efforts of these women (service users, practitioners and academics) have contributed in no small part to recent policy developments aimed at the development of gender-sensitive mental health services. In 2002 the Department of Health for England and Wales carried out a wide consultation of women service users. Powerful messages emerged both for government and mental health practitioners. Women reported that:

1. They are not listened to, nor are their views taken seriously.

2. They want access to services that are designed to empower them, promoting choice and self-determination (e.g. gender-specific or single-sex services; to choose the gender of their key worker).

3. They need mental health professionals capable of understanding the underlying causes and context of their mental distress.

4. They want recognition of their strengths and abilities as survivors.

5. They need to feel and be safe when they are receiving mental health care.

Subsequently the Department of Health launched its Women's Mental Health Strategy which aims 'to achieve a mainstream approach to gender in mental health service organisation and delivery', recognizes 'the need to listen to and involve women in planning and delivering services' and seeks 'to ensure that women feel better served by the mental health care system in terms of their individual experience' (DH, 2003). This strategy provides a framework for addressing gender inequalities in the mental health system. Moreover, from 1 April 2007, the government of England and Wales is legally required to demonstrate equity of outcome for women and men in all aspects of policy, workforce issues and service delivery under the Gender Public Sector Duty introduced as part of the Equality Bill in March 2005 (DTI, 2005). Similar legislation applies in Scotland through the Equality Act (Scottish Government, 2006).

Acknowledging that women within the voluntary sector have to a large extent already developed 'best practice', the Department of Health has emphasized the need for partnership working across statutory, voluntary and community sectors to support user-led provision. The Implementation Guidance (DH, 2003) outlines a series of key principles and objectives for commissioners and providers of mental health services to ensure the development of a gendered context for mental health care. These include:

- Listen to what women say they want and need.

- Assess women's needs, taking full account of the causes and context of their mental distress.

- Acknowledge and address the high prevalence and impact of violence and abuse in women's lives.

- Maintain women's safety – physical, sexual and psychological.

- Increase the number and range of women-only services.

- Improve services for specific groups of women, for example: women from black and minority ethnic communities, women offenders, women who self-harm, women with perinatal mental ill-health, women who experience eating disorders.

However, for these policy developments to be truly effective will require nothing short of a cultural sea-change. Some commentators are understandably cautious about the potential for such fundamental reform. In particular there are concerns that the culture of managerialism in health and social-care delivery is a potential barrier to meaningful change (Social Perspectives Network, 2005). In this context it is tempting for agencies and organizations to succumb to the pressure to achieve targets by presenting a picture of compliance with the strategy while undermining its central principles.

In addition, wider initiatives (DH, 2004) aimed at the development of integrated models of service delivery between health and social care agencies and interprofessional workforce development may inadvertently threaten the scope for developing truly gender-sensitive services. It is anticipated that there are significant benefits to be gained from joined-up approaches, such as the development of generic 'mental health practitioners' and more creative and flexible approaches to mental health care – including improvements in mental health care for women. However, while these initiatives may sound attractive in theory, they may prove problematic in practice, given the significant differences between the two professional cultures. Any potential advantages may be undermined if the new structures continue to be dominated by the traditions and culture of health with its over-reliance on the medical model – a context that has to date not served women well. Many would argue that the *social* dimension of mental health care is at risk of being lost at precisely the time when it is most urgently needed to inform the development of gender sensitivity in professional mental health education, training and practice (Tew, 2005).

There are other workforce development implications that arise from the development of gender-sensitive mental health services. The expansion of women-only services and the ability to respond to women's demands for more female professionals pose significant challenges to health and social care employers in terms of recruitment policies and practices. Furthermore, there needs to be much more attention to gender-sensitivity in mental health education and training than exists at present. Evidence drawn from the Department of Health Consultation (DH, 2002a) and elsewhere (Social Perspectives Network, 2005) points to a widespread reluctance among practitioners to treat gender and other inequalities seriously. This would suggest that the hearts and minds of mental health professionals are still not attuned to the impact of gender inequality on women's mental health, or indeed on their own attitudes and behaviour. Given the wealth of quality literature citing good practice that has amassed on this subject over the last quarter of a century, coupled with the campaigning efforts of women's groups, this state of affairs is disappointing to say the least.

Future vision

Clearly, for mental health care to become truly gender sensitive it must be informed by accurate knowledge and understanding of gender differences in women and men and how they interrelate. Possibilities for change only begin to emerge when practitioners recognize the way in which gender permeates categories of mental distress. The most obvious course of action is to shift mental health practice away from its strongly individualizing, medicalizing mould, to a frame of reference which accepts and recognizes the importance of social and material circumstances in shaping men's and women's lives and their mental health. A gendered, social model requires that women's mental health is appraised according to theoretical models that can adequately explain how 'proneness' and 'vulnerability' arise out of women's social position and their differential susceptibility and exposure to risk factors that might correlate with or lead to poor mental health outcomes. However, there should always be an awareness of individual differences (between women and men) and the way in which other dimensions of inequality may in certain circumstances transcend those of gender (for example experiences of poverty, racism, homophobia and ageism).

The inadequacies of the current system will only be remedied by organizations developing services for users that are based on thorough assessments of the users' needs and from a new understanding of men's and women's behaviour. As Sue Waterhouse (Social Perspectives Network, 2005: 93) argues, 'it won't be possible to address the needs of women and men equitably, appropriately and effectively if gender is not considered'. Women's groups, service users and mental health workers who advocate gender-sensitive services have begun to make an impact on how mental health care is being delivered. For these efforts to penetrate the mainstream requires fundamental changes in the planning and delivery of mental health services to women. Crucially, researchers, policy makers and practitioners must give legitimacy to women's views and the meanings they attach to their experiences. Without them, the evidence base, policy formation and service delivery will be fatally flawed. Ultimately, the real test of the commitment to 'mainstreaming gender' will be when women *feel and report* that they are being better served by the mental health system.

━━━━━━━━━━━━━━━━ **EDITORS' QUESTIONS** ━━━━━━━━━━━━━━━━

Issues of difference

▨ Describe the gender bias in mental health care.

▨ What gender differences occur during the lifespan?

▨ Is it a benefit or hindrance to be a female clinician on a male acute unit?

Relevance to practice

▨ How do mental health professionals communicate male issues, in your experience?

▨ In what way can female-appropriate mental health care be increased?

▨ What are the benefits of gender-specific mental health care?

Investigate

▨ How are gender-related mental health issues considered in your practice?

▨ How do you respond as a health professional to a female service user as opposed to a male service user?

▨ What power dynamics should a male clinician consider when working with a female service user?

Suggested further reading

Prior, P.M. (1999) *Gender and Mental Health*. Basingstoke: Macmillan.
Rogers, A. and Pilgrim, D. (2003) *Mental Health and Inequality*. Basingstoke: Palgrave Macmillan.

References

Barnes, D. (1997) *Older People with Mental Health Problems Living Alone: Anybody's Priority?* London: Department of Health.
Barnes, M. and Bowl, R. (2001) *Taking Over the Asylum*. Basingstoke: Palgrave Macmillan.
Barnes, M. Bowl, R. and Fisher, M. (1990) *Sectioned: Social Services and the 1983 Mental Health Act*. London: Routledge.
Bebbington, P. (1996) The origin of sex differences in depressive disorder: Bridging the gap. *International Review of Psychiatry* 8(4), 295–332.
Bebbington, P., Targosz, S. and Lewis, G. (2002) Lone mothers, social exclusion and depression. Paper presented at the Royal College of Psychiatrists Annual Conference, London.
Bracken, P. and Thomas, P. (2000) Prison wardens or mental health professionals? *Openmind* **101**: 20.
Broverman, I.K., Broverman, D.M., Clarkson, F.E., Rosenkrantz, P.S. and Volgel, S.R. (1970) Sex role stereotypes and clinical judgement of mental health. *Journal of Consulting and Clinical Psychology* **34**, 1–7.
Buck, M. (1997) The price of poverty: mental health and gender. *Critical Social Policy* **17**: 79–97.
Callahan, E.J., Bertakis, A.D., Azari, R., Helms, L.J., Robbins, J. and Miller, J. (1997) Depression in primary care: patient factors that influence recognition. *Family Medicine* **29**: 172–6.
Chesler, P. (1972) *Women and Madness*. New York: Doubleday.

Condon, J.T., Boyce, P. and Corkindale, C. (2004) The first-time fathers study: a prospective study of the mental health and wellbeing of men during the transition to parenthood. *Australian and New Zealand Journal of Psychiatry* **38**(1–2): 56–64.

Connell, R.W. (1995) *Masculinities*. Oxford: Polity Press.

Corob, A. (1987) *Working with Depressed Women*. Aldershot: Gower.

Courtenay, W.H. (2000) Constructions of masculinity and their influence on men's well-being: A theory of gender and health. *Social Science & Medicine*. **50** (10), 1385–1401.

DH (1999) *National Service Framework for Mental Health: Modern Standards and Service Models*. London: Department of Health.

DH (2000) *The NHS Plan: A Plan for Investment, A Plan for Reform*. London: Department of Health.

DH (2002a) *Women's Mental Health: into the Mainstream – Strategic Development of Mental Health Care for Women*. London: Department of Health.

DH (2002b) *National Suicide Prevention Strategy for England*. London: Department of Health.

DH (2003) *Mainstreaming Gender and Women's Mental Health: Implementation Guidance*. London: Department of Health.

DH (2004) *The Ten Essential Shared Capabilities: A Framework for the Whole of the Mental Health Workforce*. London: Department of Health.

DH (2005) *Delivering Race Equality in Mental Health Care: An Action Plan for Reform Inside and Outside Services and the Government's Response to the Independent Inquiry into the Death of David Bennett*. London: Department of Health.

Doyal, L. (2000) *Health and Work in Older Women: A Neglected Issue*. London: Pennell Initiative for Women's Health.

DTI (2005) *Public Sector Duty to Promote Gender Equality*. London: Department of Trade and Industry.

Ehrenreich, B. and English, D. (1979) *For Her Own Good: One Hundred and Fifty Years of the Experts' Advice to Women*. New York: Anchor Press.

Foucault, M. (1967) *Madness and Civilisation*. London: Tavistock.

Frosh, S. (1997) Screaming under the bridge: Masculinity, rationality and psychotherapy. In J.M. Ussher (ed.) *Body Talk: The Material and Discursive Regulation of Sexuality, Madness and Reproduction*. London: Routledge.

Glick, P., Fiske, S.T., Mladinic, A., Saiz, J.L., Abrams, D. and Masser, B. (2000) Beyond prejudice as simple antipathy: hostile and benevolent sexism across cultures. *Journal of Personality and Social Psychology* **79**(5): 763–75.

Gold, J. (1998) Gender differences in psychiatric illness and treatments: a critical review. *Journal of Nervous and Mental Diseases* **186**(12): 769–75.

Good Practices in Mental Health (1994) *Women and Mental Health: An Information Pack of Mental Health Services for Women in the United Kingdom*. London: GPMH.

GSCC (General Social Care Council) (2002) http://www.gscc.org.uk [accessed 27/09/07].

Hawton, K. (1998) Why has suicide increased in young males? *Crisis: Journal of Crisis Intervention and Suicide* **19**(3): 119–24.

Healthcare Commission (2007) *Count Me In: Results of the 2006 National Census of Inpatients in Mental Health and Learning Disability Services in England and Wales*. London: Healthcare Commission.

Henwood, M. (1998) *Ignored and Invisible? Carers' Experiences of the NHS*. London: Carers National Association.

Itzen, C. (2006) *Tackling the Health and Mental Health Effects of Domestic and Sexual Violence and Abuse*. London: Department of Health.

Kessler, R.C., McGonagle, K.A., Zhao, S., Nelson, C.B., Hughes, M., Eshleman, S., Wittchen, H.U. and Kendler, K. (1994) Lifetime and 12 month prevalence of DSM 111–R psychiatric disorders in the United States: results from the National Comorbidity Survey. *Archives of General Psychiatry* **51**: 8–19.

King, M., McKeown, E., Warner, J., Ramsay, A., Johnson, K., Cort, C., Wright, L., Blizard, R. and Davidson, O. (2003) Mental health and quality of life of gay men and lesbians in England and Wales: controlled, cross-sectional study. *British Journal of Psychiatry* **183**: 552–8.

Lester, H. and Glasby, J. (2006) *Mental Health Policy and Practice*. Basingstoke: Palgrave Macmillan.

Loring, M. and Powell, B. (1988) Gender, race and DSM111: a study of the objectivity of psychiatric diagnostic behaviour. *Journal of Health and Social Behaviour* **29**: 1–22.

McCauley, J., Kern, D.E., Kolodner, K., Dill, L., Schroeder, A.F., DeChant, Ryden, H.K., Derogatis, J. and Bass, E.B. (1997) Clinical characteristics of women with a history of child abuse: unhealed wounds. *Journal of the American Medical Association* **277**: 1362–8.

McFarlane, L. (1998) *Diagnosis: Homophobic: The Experiences of Lesbians, Gay Men and Bisexuals in Mental Health Services*. London: PACE.

McQueen, C. and Henwood, K. (2002) Young men in 'crisis': attending to the language of teenage boys' distress. *Social Science and Medicine* **55**: 1493–1509.

Mental Health Foundation (2003a) *Factsheet: Mental Health Problems*. London: Mental Health Foundation.

Mental Health Foundation (2003b) *Factsheet: Statistics on Mental Health*. London: Mental Health Foundation.

Milne, A. and Williams, J. (2003) *Women in Transition: A Literature Review of the Mental Health Risks Facing Women in Mid-Life*. London: Pennell Initiative for Women's Health.

Morris, J. (2004) *Services for People with Physical Impairments and Mental Health Support Needs*. Joseph Rowntree Foundation Findings 574. York: Joseph Rowntree Foundation.

Mullen, P., Martin, J., Anderson, J., Romans, S.E. and Herbison, P. (1993) Childhood sexual abuse and mental health in adult life. *British Journal of Psychiatry* **163**: 721–32.

Mullender, A. (1997) *Re-Thinking Domestic Violence: The Probation and Social Work Response*. London: Routledge.

NIMHE (2003) *Inside Outside: Improving Mental Health Services for Black and Minority Ethnic Communities in England*. Leeds: National Institute for Mental Health, England.

NIMHE (2004) *Celebrating our Cultures: Guidelines for Mental Health Promotion with Black and Minority Ethnic Communities*. Leeds: National Institute for Mental Health, England.

Office for National Statistics (2001) *Psychiatric Morbidity among Adults Living in Private Households, 2000*. London: HMSO.

Penfold, P.S. and Walker, G.A. (1984) *Women and the Psychiatric Paradox*. Milton Keynes: Open University Press.

Prior, P. and Hayes, B. (2001) Changing places: men replace women in mental health beds in Britain. *Social Policy and Administration* **35**(4): 397–410.

Prior, P.M. (1999) *Gender and Mental Health*. Basingstoke: Macmillan.

Resisters (2002) *Women Speak Out: Women's Experiences of Using Mental Health Services and Proposals for Change*. Leeds: Resisters.

Roberts, H. (1985) *The Patient Patients*. London: Pandora.

Rogers, A. and Pilgrim, D. (2003) *Mental Health and Inequality*. Basingstoke: Palgrave Macmillan.

Russell, D. (1995) *Women, Madness and Medicine*. Cambridge: Polity Press.

Rutter, P. (1995) *Sex in the Forbidden Zone: When Men in Power Abuse Women's Trust*. London: Aquarian.

Sayce, L. (2000) *From Psychiatric Patient to Citizen: Overcoming Discrimination and Social Exclusion*. Basingstoke: Palgrave.

SCMH (2001) *The Capable Practitioner: A Framework and List of the Practitioner Capabilities Required to Implement the National Service Framework for Mental Health*. London: Sainsbury Centre for Mental Health.

Scott, S. and Williams, J. (2001) *Report on Department of Health user/survivor consultation day*. Canterbury: Tizard Centre, University of Kent.

Scottish Government (2002) *Choose Life: A National Strategy and Action Plan to Prevent Suicide in Scotland*, Scottish Government: Edinburgh.

Scottish Government (2006) *The Equality Act 2006*, Scottish Government: Edinburgh.

Sheppard, M. (1991) General practice, social work and mental health sections: the social control of women. *British Journal of Social Work* **21**, 663–83.

Sheppard, M. (2002) Mental health and social justice: gender, race and psychological consequences of unfairness. *British Journal of Social Work* **32**, 779–97.

Showalter, E. (1987) *The Female Malady: Women, Madness and English Culture, 1830–1980*. London: Virago.

Simoni-Wastila, L. (2000) The use of abusable prescription drugs: the role of gender. *Journal of Women's Health and Gender Based Medicine* **9**, 289–97.

Singleton, N., Maung, N.A., Cowie, A., Sparks, J., Bumpstead, R. and Meltzer, H. (2002) *Mental Health of Carers*. London: TSO.

Social Perspectives Network (2005) *SPN Paper 7. Women and Mental Health: turning rhetoric into reality – sharing practice perspectives and strategies for action on women's mental health*. London: Social Perspectives Network.

Soliday, E., McCluskey-Fawcett, K. and O'Brien, M. (1999) Postpartum affect and depressive symptoms in mothers and fathers. *American Journal of Orthopsychiatry* **69**, 30–8.

Spurrell, M., Hatfield, B. and Perry, A. (2003) Characteristics of patients presenting for emergency psychiatric assessment at an English hospital. *Psychiatric Services* **54**(2): 240–45.

Stoppard, J.M. (1997) Women's bodies, women's lives and depression: towards a reconciliation of material and discursive accounts. In: J.M. Ussher (ed.) *Body Talk: The Material and Discursive Regulation of Sexuality, Madness and Reproduction*. London: Routledge.

Stoppe, G., Sandholzer, H. and Huppertz, C. (1999) Gender differences in the recognition of depression in old age. *Maturitas* **32**, 205–12.

Tew, J. (ed.) (2005) *Social Perspectives in Mental Health: Developing Social Models to Understand and Work with Mental Distress*. London: Jessica Kingsley.

Thompson, N. (2001) *Anti-discriminatory Practice* (3rd edn). Basingstoke: Palgrave Macmillan.

Ussher, J.M. (1991) *Women's Madness: Misogyny or Mental Illness?* Hemel Hempstead: Harvester Wheatsheaf.

Warren, L.W. (1983) Male intolerance of depression: a review with implications for psychotherapy. *Clinical Psychology Review* **3**, 147–56.

Wetzel, J.W. (2000) Women and mental health: a global perspective. *International Social Work* **34**(2): 205–15.

White, R. (2002) Social and political aspects of men's health. *Health* **6**(3): 267–85.

Williams, J., Watson, G., Smith, H., Copperman, J. and Wood, D. (1993) *Purchasing Effective Mental Health Services for Women: A Framework for Action*. Canterbury: University of Kent.

Wilson, M. (2001) Black women and mental health: working toward inclusive mental health services. *Feminist Review* **68**, 34–51.

Wood, D. (1993) *The Power of Words: Uses and Abuses of Talking Treatments*. London: MIND.

Wood, D. and Copperman, J. (1996) Sexual harassment and assault in psychiatric services. In R. Perkins, Z. Nadirshaw, J. Copperman and C. Andrews (eds) *Women in Context: Good Practices in Mental Health Services for Women*. London: Good Practices in Mental Health.

WHO (2000) *Women's Mental Health: An Evidence-Based Review*. Geneva: World Health Organization.

WHO (2001) *Gender Disparities in Mental Health*. Geneva: World Health Organization.

WHO (2002) *Gender and Mental Health*. Geneva: World Health Organization.

7

The Lifespan

David Pilgrim, Anne Rogers and Robert Tummey

BRIEF CHAPTER OUTLINE

Exploring the lifespan, the authors offer a view that considers a range of issues within an age-related context. Quite simply, the chapter addresses mental illness from birth to death. Opening with antenatal life, inequalities at the outset are detailed, leading into infancy. Within the childhood section, an overview is given on attachment and psychodynamic theory. Adolescence is then explored as the transition from childhood to adulthood, a vulnerable period of potential dysfunctional withdrawal. Middle adulthood highlights the time of responsibility and competence. Any withdrawal from this is more obvious than in any other stage of the lifespan. Older adulthood concludes the chapter, identifying disparity between the mental health needs of older people and the services they receive.

Introduction

A lifespan approach to mental health highlights that human existence in a basic sense is fixed for us all. We are conceived, we are born, we develop and then we die after a variable period of time. The events within and between these stages and even the length of time involved are shaped and influenced by social factors. A lifespan approach sensitizes us to what happens at a moment in time (synchronic factors) and across time (diachronic factors). It also invites us to examine the contention surrounding forms of determinism (what causes mental health problems) and the biopsychosocial consequences of mental health problems. With this complexity in mind, this chapter will commence from antenatal life through to old age.

Antenatal life: inequalities at the outset

The extent to which mental health problems can be attributed to genetic disposition has been fraught with controversy. The psychiatric profession, since its inception in the middle of the nineteenth century, has been linked to a strong advocacy of genetic determination. During the twentieth century this genetic viewpoint remained in the ascendancy and it still resonates strongly today. For example, even in diagnoses where biological aetiology remains assumed but actually mysterious, such as 'schizophrenia' and 'bipolar disorder', some genetic risk is evident but it does not follow neat patterns.

In the case of the diagnosis of bipolar disorder, this is twice as likely in first-degree relatives of those already diagnosed (Gelder, Mayou and Cowen, 2001). This still means that the great majority (75–92 per cent) of relatives do *not* receive the diagnosis. The lack of neat patterning suggests polygenic inheritance – several genes in some form of yet-to-be-discerned interaction (Sanders, Detera-Wadleigh and Gershon, 1999). This point is important because bipolar disorder is put forward by biological psychiatrists as the most hereditable of all mental illnesses. Moreover, these biodeterminists have to concede from their data (mainly from twin and other family studies (Kendler, Neale and Kessler, 1992)) that this genetic link is highly problematic in unipolar depression. In the latter there are twice as many females as men diagnosed, even though no sex-linked genetic pattern is discernible. The female preponderance has to be accounted for by non-genetic effects.

The rhetorical overstatement of the genetic case dates back to the eugenic roots of psychiatry. Eugenics, the pseudo-science of human improvement, was common and respectable in all Eurocentric cultures in the mid-nineteenth century. Psychiatry was a particular beneficiary of this conventional wisdom of the time because it was not clear how madness and misery could be claimed as medical conditions. The answer lay in asserting that mental disorders were hereditable brain disorders, ensuring medical authority over madness. Even when the links with Nazi race science were clearly established in the 1930s, post-war psychiatry still incorporated and utilized its hereditarian findings (Marshall, 1990). However, after over a century of research into the genetics of mental disorder, even biological psychiatrists tend now to the more tentative position that their favoured candidates ('schizophrenia' and 'bipolar disorder') reflect an inherited *predisposition* towards 'major mental disorder', rather than direct heredity.

There have been two dangers with the professionally expedient use of genetic arguments. The first is that they have diverted the attention of psychiatry from a robust understanding of psychosocial antecedents and consequences of mental health problems. The profession became over-reliant on heredity in its theorizing and training (Kemker and Khadivi, 1995) and so it has not been able to deliver on its rhetoric of biopsychosocial or holistic assessments and treatment of service users (Moncrieff and Crawford, 2001). It has also been unable to engage efficiently and consistently with the social sciences, to the detriment of both service users and the wider multidisciplinary effort to research all aspects of mental health (Pilgrim and Rogers, 2005).

The second danger is the opposite side of the same coin. The strong environmentalist reaction, to what has been more professional ideology than medical science, can divert us from taking demonstrable genetic risk seriously. For example, there are some disabling conditions, which are clearly inherited. The best example is Huntington's Disease (HD), where the precise genetic source can be identified and the risk to offspring calculated. Apart from cognitive deficits, people with HD manifest a range of manic, depressive and paranoid symptoms. This disorder and other inherited ones affecting mental states, such as porphyria and turberose sclerosis, are rare. However, they remind us that the understandable suspicion of biological psychiatry and its enmeshment historically with eugenics may unhelpfully divert us from understanding some serious mental health problems.

When we shift our attention from genetic to congenital effects then we are immediately in the domain of environmental determinism, even if the latter is antenatal in relevance and impact. Thus 'biological' cannot logically be equated with 'genetic' as there is an important biological dimension to our *environment*. The elision between genetic determination and environmental biological determination is not uncommon in biomedical reasoning (Guze, 1989).

Alongside this error is the assumption that biology means pathology to be understood by medical science. But given that *all* behaviour is underpinned by a biological substrate, this logic is flawed. Biology (in its genetic and environmental aspects) makes a contribution to behavioural diversity in a population. The labelling of some behaviour as problematic is primarily a social judgement which medicine codifies. To say that depression is a biological condition is true in the sense that happiness, curiosity and boredom are also biological conditions. But biological does not mean pathological. The latter is socially agreed, not naturally given.

Infancy and childhood: trust and attachment

The foetus, then, with no inherited or congenital disadvantage, encounters the challenge of birth. Early life after birth has been explored most extensively in variants of a form of psychology (psychoanalysis), which is inherently interested, because of its developmental focus, in the type and quality of relationships in early childhood. In particular, those psychoanalysts who modified Freud's original emphasis upon the Oedipus complex (the child desiring the parent of the opposite sex and learning to rescind these desires) emphasized pre-Oedipal and even pre-verbal experiences. This group of 'object-relations' theorists, including Balint, Winnicott, Fairbairn and Guntrip, argued that the developmental challenge for the infant is to find a suitable balance between fusion and separation with their caregiver (depicted at that time as the mother–child bond) in order to grow confidently as a separate individual. For example, here Winnicott talks of the early joining and separating of 'the baby and the mother when the mother's love, displayed as human reliability, does in fact give the baby a sense of trust, or of confidence in the environmental factor' (1967: 372).

For Winnicott this primary or primitive form of relating leads to the baby internalizing a sense of trust when the care is good. His preferred phrase was 'good-enough' because imperfect trust also creates a space for the baby to struggle and separate from the mother – to individuate. His use of the term 'environmental factor' suggests that from a psychoanalytical perspective our general trust in our environment relies on early maternal trustworthiness. Some psychoanalysts suggested that the brief interlude between being safely in the womb and being held safely outside it offered the first major risk of threat to trust in the infant – 'birth trauma' (Rank, 1929).

For Winnicott and other object relations theorists, the emphasis is on mutual empathy. The baby innately trusts the mother and the mother provides a safe physical and emotional environment for the infant to grow. By implication, neglect or abuse during infancy can impair the person's capacity to trust the world generally. This would create intense anxiety, which could be experienced as paranoia or chaotic madness.

Likewise Fairbairn (1952) argued that the baby was not 'pleasure-seeking' (the classic Freudian assumption) but 'object-seeking'. The term 'object' here may appear odd, as it actually refers to 'person', but it is based on the assumption that the pre-verbal and, by definition, egocentric, baby, at its stage of development seeks to relate to its caregivers but does not recognize their existence as whole separate human beings (yet). Support from this idea comes from the study of feral children who have been raised by animals. They seek the care of these other species and adopt their habits. The children survive, albeit in a pre-verbal state. In other words, the infant seeks connection and attachment but does not recognize, or have a reflective sense of, the full nature of his or her carer.

These psychoanalytical ideas were joined in the 1950s by evidence from a different direction-ethology (the study of animal behaviour and its adaptive value for the preservation of a species). Bowlby (1969) was a psychoanalyst who drew heavily on the work of ethology to support his theories about attachment. The most famous and oft quoted to, and by, students of psychology is the work of Harlow. The latter studied the attachment and feeding behaviour of baby rhesus monkeys. In one version of his experiment (Harlow and Zimmerman, 1959) the monkeys were fed on demand from one of two models – one was simply a wire structure with a feeding bottle; the other was covered with a cloth. The babies preferred the latter and spent most of their time with it, whether or not they were being fed. Moreover, this preference extended to wanting the cloth model even when its milk had run out and milk was still available from the wire model (Harlow, 1961).

The conclusion drawn here is that the infant's basic need to attach and relate to others precedes and is even more basic than food seeking. A further implication of this primary desire for attachment in humans (and other primates) is that our tendency towards healthy and unhealthy forms of relationship may be determined very early in life (Bowlby, 1953). Indeed, it is so early in life (enacted immediately from the springboard of an instinctive predisposition) that our later moral entitlement to receive, and obligation to give, trust, as rule following behaviour which is codified in and learned via language, may be an elaboration of this basic tendency.

Psychologists from a variety of theoretical perspectives agree that neglect and abuse in childhood are not good for a person's mental health. Causality is always seen as multiple, however, and includes genetic vulnerability and social stress within and around a family of origin. What is clear is that privation (withholding care), deprivation (taking care away or providing inadequate care) and abuse (whether it is emotional, physical or sexual) significantly increase the probability of many mental health problems both in childhood and later in adulthood (Browne, Davies and Stratton, 1988).

The broad claims made by Bowlby about the risks of failed benign attachment or its loss in infancy and childhood appear to be borne out empirically (Bifulco, Harris and Brown, 1992; Cichetti, Toch and Lynch, 1995). For example, abuse in early infancy predicts psychotic symptoms such as hallucinations, delusions and thought disorder (Read *et al.*, 2003; Whitfield *et al.*, 2005). Abuse in childhood also predicts outpatient attendance at psychiatric facilities and is significantly linked to specific symptoms such as attempted suicide, revictimization in adulthood, substance misuse, sleep disturbances, panic attacks, depression, sexual problems and fear of others (Briere and Runtz 1988; Stein *et al.* 1988). Sexually abused children may also be at increased risk of going on themselves to become adult abusers (Becker, 1988; Dimock, 1988).

Parents who are overcritical and perfectionistic increase the risk of their children presenting later with social phobia or obsessive-compulsive problems (Stakettee and Frost, 1998). Children who grow up feeling the need to look after their parents (role reversal) are more likely to develop chronic generalized anxiety (Borkovec and Newman, 1998). The safety and reliability of early family life makes the difference between adults suffering adversity surviving or becoming depressed (Brown and Harris, 1978; Brown, Haris and Hepworth, 1995).

Early deprivation and abuse also predict a proclivity for abusing substances in adulthood and, in the case of physical abuse, it increases the probability of violent acting-out (assaults on strangers and domestic violence). Indeed, it is difficult to find a form of mental health problem which is unaffected by negative childhood experiences, though debates still rage about the proportion of influence it has (compared to biological predisposition and one-off severe traumas or cumulative social stress). Moreover, the biological, psychological and social systems interact and influence one another in multiple and circular ways. It is worth noting that the term 'biological' here may not always mean 'genetic' because the biological environment affects the growing brain post-partum. In turn, the child's behaviour starts to affect his or her social opportunities at a very early age.

The early environment affects the developing personality of the child – its stable psychological characteristics in later life. When these stable features are dysfunctional the person can acquire the label of 'personality disorder'. The two most common diagnoses given to prisoners who are deemed to be personality disordered are 'borderline' and 'antisocial personality disorder'. In the first of these diagnoses (given more to women than men) there is a consistent pattern of histories of sustained verbal, physical or sexual abuse in childhood (Widiger and Trull, 1994). Physical abuse is a recurring pattern of those with a diagnosis of antisocial personality disorder. Retrospective accounts identify a pattern of oppositional behaviour and violence from a young age.

What these offenders have in common is a marked egocentricity. With this comes a lack of empathy for others or at least an indifference to their rights and feelings. Other people only represent an opportunity for their needs being met – they are not recognized as having needs of their own, with an equal entitlement to have these needs met. At the centre of those with a personality disorder is egocentricity and a lack of mutuality, respect and trust in relation to other human beings. Others are used as sources of gratification and their needs and rights are not respected (or they are manipulated in a callous or instrumental manner for selfish ends). As a consequence of this amoral position, actions are inevitably judged by others to be offensive and incorrigible. Sustained egocentricity (rather than the transitory selfish moments and specific weaknesses of all humans) is inherently asocial and amoral. However, it grows in moral, social and political significance when it acquires the extraordinary powers enjoyed by leaders in society. This point cues the next section.

Adolescence: regression and fixation

Primary socialization highlights two important points about mental health status. First, learning to obey rules, being exposed to stressors in childhood and controlling our emotions come at a price; we are all, to some degree, neurotic. Second, the roots of many expressions of madness, sadness and badness can be found during early development. When the young person is faced with the challenge of the transition from childhood to adulthood, they enter this vulnerable period with varying degrees of self-confidence or 'ego-strength'. At this juncture, a refusal of, or inhibition about, the adult role (with its emphasis on rationality, responsibility and comfort with external reality) increases the chances of forms of dysfunctional withdrawal. Psychosis and eating disorders are both expressions of the latter. The anxious imagination can be confused with reality (delusions) and imagery can be confused with perception (hallucinations). Analogously, the adolescent anorexic puts herself (and less often himself) developmentally in suspended animation.

One of the most controversial questions in current debates about mental health is the nature of madness (Bentall 1990, 2005; Boyle, 1991). Psychiatrists are divided or uncertain about the cause or causes of such symptoms. Many argue that 'schizophrenia' is a genetically programmed 'time bomb', which explodes in adolescence, disturbing the functioning of the brain and the person. Others follow the view of Winnicott (1958) noted earlier that it is an environmental disease, resulting from poor maternal care in the first year of life, leaving the person psychologically weak and without a secure sense of self. Adolescence marks a time when the person's sense of identity and capacity for independence are under scrutiny and strain, making them vulnerable to psychotic breakdown and regression to the psychological chaos of early infancy. Others tried to render schizophrenic behaviour intelligible within the confused and confusing communication pattern of the patient's family (Laing and Esterson, 1964).

The questions begged for sociologists about schizophrenia are mainly about how the diagnosis is negotiated or ascribed. Coulter (1973) argues that focusing on debates about aetiology obscures the ways in which madness emerges in its social context. It is actually first negotiated in the lay area and then it is professionally confirmed with a diagnosis. Coulter focuses on everyday expectations of normality and social competence. For example, in relation to hallucinations he argues that to maintain our credibility in a social group there has to be a consensus about what our senses detect around us. In most contexts, if a person sees or hears something which others do not, then their social credibility and group membership are jeopardized. However, it is possible in certain contexts that such idiosyncratic capacities might raise rather than diminish their credibility and group status. The Christian mystic and some African medicine men are actually expected to have extraordinary visions to have credibility in their role. Their mandate may rest on having these abnormal experiences.

In some cultures where hallucinations are valued positively, the bodily circumstances that increase the probability of their occurrence (such as fasting, fatigue and drug-taking) are often contrived deliberately. Al-Issa (1977) notes that, in western society, hallucinations offend rational norms. Most of us suppress idiosyncratic perceptions because we learn that they are not positively valued. The person with 'schizophrenia', by contrast, makes the mistake of, or is driven to, acting upon their idiosyncratic experiences.

Community surveys indeed point to estimates of between 10 per cent and 50 per cent of the 'normal' population who hallucinate – psychotic experiences are on a continuum; they are not in separate populations, one ill and the other well (Tien, 1991; van Os *et al.*, 2000). Thus, atypical idiosyncratic perceptions are not intrinsically pathological.

Whether hallucinations are deemed to indicate a gift or a defect depends on the social context being studied. Likewise, weird speech patterns are highly valued in those Christian sects which celebrate the ability to 'speak in tongues' (or 'glossolalia') (Bentall and Pilgrim, 1993; Szasz, 1992). Outside these sects, in everyday western life, they may be taken to be an offence to rational discourse and so encourage attributions of mad talk or, in psychiatric terms, 'thought disorder'.

Some recent sociological accounts of madness have gone beyond Coulter's point about the attribution of unintelligibility and explored the meaning of service users' narratives as a pathway to understanding how people cope with a psychiatric diagnosis. When a young person receives a diagnosis of 'schizophrenia' then they reflect on their pre-existing sense of self, but these reflections on identity are not always negative (Dinos *et al.*, 2004). This ambiguity can be contrasted with the tendency of relatives of service users seeing them as being 'lost' to the illness (Barham and Hayward, 1991).

The diagnosis of 'schizophrenia' predominates in young adulthood. That is, when role expectations based on rational rule-following and goal orientation are highlighted. It is the time of life when the rationality of work and parenting, competency and responsibility are demanded of, and by, those involved. The person with 'schizophrenia' defies or violates these expectations about dealing with external reality and adopting conduct appropriate for the adult work role. This point takes us to the next section.

Middle adulthood: workers and parents

Adulthood has been described as 'mediating two stages of life, best expressed in the story of a dying man. As he lay with his eyes closed, his wife whispered the names of all family members present. "And who," he suddenly asked, sitting up abruptly, "who is minding the store?"' (Erikson, 1998). This expresses the spirit and responsibility of adulthood and illustrates the adult position. It also demonstrates the process of attempting to control one's own environment. As an adult, attempts to attain such control and choice in life are a driving force. Should this pursuit be halted at any point through mental illness, the position of responsibility and control can become less attainable. Therefore, within mental health services, while health is the concern of the practitioner, it is also the responsibility of the service user. Assistance and encouragement promote partnership, but should never be dominated by the professional (Tummey and Smojkis, 2005). It is imperative that the service user's responsibility is considered and any contractual obligations such as advanced directives are honoured (Minett *et al.*, 2005).

Adult women are more prone than men to be diagnosed with 'common mental disorders', though the reasons for this are by no means clear (Rhodes and Goering, 1998). It may reflect a difference in stress, with patriarchy protecting men and oppressing women. It may be an artefact of service contact (most diagnoses of common mental disorders occur in primary care, and women attend the latter much more frequently than men). It may also reflect gender bias in diagnosis. (For a discussion of this ambiguity see Gove, 1984; Busfield, 1988 and Nazroo, Edwards and Brown, 1998.)

For many adult women, the impact of domestic abuse is a major cause of difficulty for both physical and mental health. The behaviour that constitutes domestic violence is wide-ranging, including threats and intimidation, physical assault, humiliation, withholding money, sexual abuse, rape, denying physical freedom or medical care and belittling. Predominantly, men perpetrate incidents of domestic violence and abuse against women. Lethal consequences occur frequently. Statistics for England and Wales show that half of all adult female homicide victims are killed by a current or former male partner and have estimated that one woman dies every three days as a result of domestic violence (Home Office, 2000). Domestic abuse has a devastating effect on the mental health of women and needs to be the business of all health professionals (Tummey, 2003).

Navigating any life experiences can take its toll on the adult. The impact of several milestones in life becomes a contributing factor to the mental health of the individual who may be having difficulty tolerating the experience. This includes work and attempts to provide for oneself or one's family, getting a better financial deal or conditions, maintaining self-esteem, feeling a purpose in attending the process of work, social context and so on. If unemployed, then a different set of mental health concerns emerge. Adverse effects of unemployment on family life include a higher risk of domestic violence, divorce and separation, unwanted pregnancy, increased perinatal and infant mortality, poorer infant growth and increased health-service use (Smith, 1987).

Work also brings with it both threats to mental health and positive opportunities. Unemployment is bad for mental health, but so is poorly paid and insecure employment. For a person with mental illness, the very real prospect of unemployment is rather inevitable. This further compounds the social exclusion experienced, reducing social contact and alienation from mainstream society, defined by Sayce as:

> the interlocking and mutually compounding problems of impairment, discrimination, diminished social role, lack of economic and social participation and disability. Among the factors at play are lack of status, joblessness, lack of opportunities to establish a family, small or non-existent social networks, compounding race and other discriminations, repeated rejection and consequent restriction to hope and expectation.
>
> (Sayce, 2000: 9)

Here the role of the adult carer is a significant one. For the carer of an adult with mental illness there are many losses to endure, including loss of previous identity, routine, enjoyment, socializing, financial security, autonomy, parental control, development and order, to name but a few. Often carers are isolated and join support groups as a replacement social network. Both the physical and mental health of the carer can suffer. Indeed, the response of the carer to the family member with mental illness is an important mediator of the illness outcome (Butzlaff and Hooley, 1998). Reactions can include over-optimistic expectation of a return to previous stability. When not realized, this can lead to criticism and attempts to compensate for impairments by taking over their social roles, what has been referred to as 'expressed emotion' (Repper and Perkins, 2003). It is important to recognize that expressed emotion and over-involvement are equally prevalent among mental health practitioners (Repper and Perkins, 2003).

This may bring into question the competence of the adult and their ability to give consent. Within English 'Tort' law, 'trespass to the person' is committed when there is direct intentional application of force upon a person. The major defence against Tort is consent (Kirby *et al.*, 2004). Service users can give consent verbally or in writing, but it can also be implied (as when attending a doctor's appointment for examination). To be valid, consent must be free of coercion and the person must be mentally competent.

The competent person is one who has provided knowledgeable consent to treatment. Kennedy and Grubb (1994: 127) propose that 'the doctor has an obligation to educate and ascertain whether the person has understood the facts ... If they do not, then the doctor does not have informed consent.' If the person is unable to give valid consent then guardianship, power of attorney or welfare attorney may be required. If no provision is in place, then courts take the decision based on the premise that treatment is in the best interests of the person as judged by a responsible body of medical opinion. (See Mental Capacity Act – DH, 2005 – and Adult with Incapacity Act – Scottish Government, 2000.)

Also, within adulthood there can be the unenvious position of nonconformity to societal norms and subsequent exclusion. This is often a position held by people with mental illness who may not work, have no family and who are viewed with suspicion. It is also a position occupied by people of a different race, culture, sexual orientation, values, class and socioeconomic status who conduct their lives in contrast to the perceived norms. The removed position is generally held by the adult and is more obvious than in any other stage of the lifespan.

These points highlight that the life course brings with it negative and positive social forces that affect mental health. All lives are also saturated until death by other influences, particularly race, class and gender. The tendency of 'mental health services' (a euphemism for services dedicated to the management of mental *disorder*) to be the focus of 'mental health policy' (another euphemism) is important. Even though studies of overall mental health status suggest that the highest prevalence of problems is in children and the very old, these demographic groups have less state funding for specialist services. This is politically significant and highlights that the state's priorities about regulating forms of deviance that are framed as mental disorder or mental health problems focus on people of *working age with parental responsibilities.*

Thus 'mental health services' reflect a wing of the state's apparatus of control. Work and family life constitute a moral and economic order that requires correction when and if it becomes dysfunctional or disordered. This status is rarely acknowledged by politicians or by many mental health professionals who tend to prefer a paternalistic discourse of 'treating illness' or 'responding to needs'. The overall focus is on deficits and dysfunction and a primary aim to reduce such deficits, namely symptoms (Repper and Perkins 2003). User-led research conducted by Faulkner and Layzell (2000) found that there is a 'series of common themes in what people sought from mental health services. The removal or reduction of deficits or symptoms was not one of them.'

Old age: leaving the labour market and biological decline

The material reality of becoming old is evident to us all (even to the most radical social constructivist). The prospect of our three score years and ten, give or take a range of years according to our sex, class and global context, focuses the mind of all of us as we grow older. No one lives forever. In the years prior to death in old age, health risks multiply. And old age brings with it particular threats to mental health. Dementia is the most obvious cultural motif of old-age mental ill-health. But depression is actually much more common in older people than dementia. Also, dementia is not limited to older people but can occur in younger people as well. Not only do we find forms of dementia in middle-aged people, but some much younger people can be vulnerable to particular forms of it (such as CJD from BSE infection).

There is a secondary mental health impact of dementia – it affects informal carers (Morris, Morris and Britton, 1988). Stress reactions are common in this group of carers, although some other studies highlight positive as well as negative psychological features of the caring role (Orbell, Hopkins and Gillies, 1993). In those with advanced dementia, direct physical care is demanded in a way which is usually not implied in younger people with diagnoses such as schizophrenia.

Whereas the prevalence of dementia is about 5 per cent in the over-65s, rising to just below 20 per cent for those over 80, depression is much more common in the younger age-band of older people. Community surveys have indicated prevalence rates for depression of between 5 per cent in Edinburgh (Maule, Milne and Williamson, 1984) and 26 per cent in Newcastle (Kay, Beamish and Roth, 1964) for people over 65. More typically, studies quote rates of 11–15 per cent (Copeland *et al.*, 1987).

Around 2 per cent of the UK population of over-65s is in residential care. In this population, the prevalence of depression rises dramatically. A metropolitan survey of 12 residential care homes for older people revealed that around 40 per cent of the residents were depressed (Mann, Graham and Ashby, 1984). Surveys in Australia (Snowden and Donnelly, 1986) found one-third of the residents depressed and a similar survey finding was reported from Italy (Spagnoli *et al.*, 1986). Mild depression is more common in older women and it is also more prevalent in older men and women suffering from physical illnesses (Brayne and Ames, 1988).

The degree of association between depression and physical ill-health is shown by a study of 100 people referred over a 30-month period to a older adult service with depression (Dover and McWilliam, 1992). The authors found that only 3 per cent of the men and 20 per cent of the women patients were physically healthy. The rest had a variety of serious conditions including cancer, cardiovascular disease, arthritis, deafness and respiratory problems. Sixty-five per cent of the sample were suffering from 'multiple illness'. Moreover, many of the treatments for some of these physical disorders are known to cause or amplify depressed mood, suggesting an iatrogenic component in this group of depressed physically ill people. The association of depression with physical illness in old age is highlighted in the review of several studies of non-psychiatric in-patients, which concluded that only one in five recover from their lowered mood state before death (Cole and Bellavance, 1997). Suicide rates also increase in the older age group, especially in men.

How is the data understood from psychiatric epidemiology of depression in older people? Starting with the very high prevalence of depression in residential homes, there are three possible explanations, which are not mutually exclusive. First, *those selected to enter these homes* have been deemed by relatives or professionals already to be in poor mental health, or vulnerable because of their lonely and under-supported home conditions (hence their referral to the homes).

Secondly, the *under-stimulating environment* of these homes may create apathy and morbid introspection (in the jargon of psychiatry, 'dysphoria'). This has led some psychiatrists of old age to suggest the homes may contain a number of people who are not 'clinically depressed' but who rather suffer from environmentally induced dysphoria, which may dissipate within a more stimulating care regime. Such a construction on the data assumes that there are clear demarcations to be made between clinical descriptions of 'true' depression and other experiences, such as apathy, anomie, listlessness, sad brooding and so on. Some other 'psycho-geriatricians' have pointed out that, in practice, in most cases of sad old people it is not easy to pigeonhole them as being 'ill' or 'not ill' (Murphy *et al.*, 1988).

Thirdly, being moved to a residential facility is disruptive, entails a loss of previous surroundings and marks a loss of personal control or autonomy. This *imposed disruption and loss* may have a depressing impact on the old person.

Turning to the community data on depression in old age, there are other explanations that could be offered for depression in old people who are not in residential care. For instance, the probability of *physical illness increases with age*, rendering older people particularly vulnerable to depression (Post, 1969). However, Blaxter (1990), investigating the self-reported physical and mental well-being of people across the lifespan, found that overall psychosocial well-being improves relatively in old age. This could be partially accounted for by the lower expectations of life quality in older people, leading to an underreporting of distress. Another factor is the dramatic improvement in the self-reported psychosocial well-being of better-off people living in more comfortable surroundings.

Relationships that have accumulated during a life are lost. Spouses, friends and siblings die off around a surviving older person, making them prone to *the aggregating effect of grief.* Depression in old age may be understandable in whole or part as the impact of cumulative grief.

Another social vulnerability factor is *material adversity*. In a community study of life events preceding depression in old age, Murphy (1982) found that poorer people who had experienced housing and financial difficulties were more depressed than better-off older people. Blaxter (1990) found that the psychosocial well-being of older people varied significantly with socioeconomic status. Social classes 1 and 2 improved with age overall but those in social classes 4 and 5 deteriorated. The lower mental health scores in very old age remind us of the inverted U pattern across the lifespan. In western societies we attain our optimal mental health in later life (average at 63 years) before starting to risk declining mental health ratings (Wade and Cairney, 1997). Basically, older people who are better off and can remain fit for their age tend to enjoy good mental health.

Another factor is the *role of supportive and confiding relationships*. Lowenthal (1965) found, like Brown and Harris (1978) in their study of younger women, that the presence of a stable confiding relationship protected against depression in old age. She also found that those who are most vulnerable are old people who try to form relationships but fail, not those who have coped alone throughout life. In her community survey Murphy (1982) found that 30 per cent of those without a confiding relationship were depressed. However, given that 70 per cent of this group were not depressed, a multi-factorial model of vulnerability and protective factors seems to be indicated (as with Brown and Harris, 1978). This reminds us that reductionist accounts (i.e. single-factor explanations) about mental ill-health are as suspect as those in the study of physical health.

A final depressogenic factor to consider is that of *elder abuse*. Eastman (1984) suggested that estimates of abused older people in the USA vary from 600,000 to over a million. As with the abuse of children, prevalence and incidence are difficult to estimate accurately, given that abusers will typically deny the act. When the abuse is perpetrated by paid carers, then their job is at stake, as well as their reputation. Estimates of abuse rates in Scandinavia vary from 8 per cent to 17 per cent of older victims across Denmark, Sweden and Finland. In one of the Swedish samples 12 per cent of the relatives of older people admitted violence (Hydle, 1993).

Some have extended the notion of elder abuse to medical neglect and iatrogenic disease in hospitalized older people (Gorbien, Bishop and Beers, 1992). This iatrogenic impact arises from, for example, poor skin care, poor infection control, failure to make accurate physical diagnoses, leaving frail elderly people at risk of falls, and inadequate dietary provision. The immediate and long-term negative psychological impact of abuse and neglect are difficult to ascertain but it is self-evident that sexual or emotional abuse or physical violence against, or neglect of, old people will not enhance their mental health.

Service provision for older people is skewed towards dementia care. However, recently there has been some effort to provide for older people experiencing depression in primary care. Treatment regimes for depression seem to mirror those being provided for groups of younger people experiencing depression, which focus mainly on the use of antidepressants (Baldwin *et al.*, 2003). More normalized activities might offer psychological amelioration. For example, gardens have been identified as a 'therapeutic landscape'. Gardening activities have been found to offer comfort and opportunity for emotional and spiritual renewal in old age. Communal gardening activity on allotments has been found to contribute to psychological well-being via the provision of a mutually supportive environment which enhances emotional well-being through combating social isolation, contributing to the development of social networks and enhancing the quality of life and emotional well-being of older people (Milligan, Gatrell and Bingley, 2004).

Conclusion

The risk of mental health problems varies throughout the lifespan. Despite the cliché of the mid-life crisis, the most vulnerable groups are children and very old people. The focus of investment in specialist mental health services for people of working age is not because this group is particularly vulnerable to mental health problems; in fact the reverse is the case, with our best mental health on average being enjoyed in those middle years. That investment says more about the need of the state and a wider moral order in society to regulate work and family life – hence those of working age raising children warrant extra scrutiny and social control. Moreover, this does not imply that a corrective social policy to improve the mental health of the young and the very old would be about more investment in specialized services (though that might make a positive contribution).

Discerning a social pattern about mental health does not logically require that more 'services' are resourced to mirror that pattern. For example, effective policies to reduce abuse and neglect in childhood are far more important than special pleading for more money for child mental health services. The latter would be ameliorative, not preventative.

As was clear in the descriptions given of the psychosocial context of these vulnerable age cohorts, improvements in mental health would arise from non-service factors. In particular, the reduction of family stressors and the increase in the availability of benign, supportive intimate relationships are critical in maximizing quality of life, self-esteem and self-confidence. Through such constructive and supportive relationships come interdependency rather than dependency or isolation and a *raison d'être* rather than *anomie*. Without positive relationships most people become unhappy and have little reason to live.

While this truism needs to be stated, caution is also warranted. The centrality of positive relationships for mental health and the obverse, the avoidance of abusive or neglectful ones, can generate its own form of reductionism. The possibility of benign supportive relating, the 'psycho' part of the compound notion of 'psychosocial', is shaped by the wide implied 'social' part of the compound. To be powerless by dint of age is included in the latter, as are implications about being poor, poorly educated and of course female rather than male (though arguments about whether women are or are not differentially vulnerable to mental health problems persist). Any understanding of shifting risks to mental health during the lifespan has to take into account other social variables, especially race, class and gender, which separately and together create differences in both the prevalence and type of mental health problems.

EDITORS' QUESTIONS

Issues of difference

- In what ways would middle age impact on a female service user?
- How can the older service user's sexual expression be ensured?
- How are the cultural needs of adults catered for in mental health care?

Relevance to practice

- How do mental health professionals assess age-related need in older age?
- How can age stereotypes be confronted by different disciplines?
- What are the age-related issues in adolescent mental health?

Investigate

- How would you respond to an older female person as opposed to a young male?
- What are the key elements for identifying and preventing discrimination of age within mental health services?
- What are the main issues for the various ages of the lifespan?

Suggested further reading

Bentall, R.P. (2005) *Madness Explained*. London: Penguin.
Erikson, E.H. (1998) *The Life Cycle Completed*. London: Norton.

References

Al-Issa, I. (1977) Social and cultural aspects of hallucinations. *Psychological Bulletin* **84**: 570–87.
Baldwin, R.C., Anderson, D., Black, S., Evans, S., Jones, R., Wilson, K. and Iliffe, S. (2003) Guidelines for the management of late-life depression in primary care. *International Journal of Geriatric Psychiatry* **18**(9): 829–38.
Barham, P. and Hayward, R. (1991) *From the Mental Patient to the Person*. London: Routledge.
Becker, J.V. (1988) The effects of child sexual abuse on adolescent sexual offenders. In: G.E. Wyatt and G.J. Powell (eds) *Lasting Effects of Child Sexual Abuse*. New York: Sage.
Bentall, R.P. (2005) *Madness Explained*. London: Penguin.
Bentall, R.P. (ed.) (1990) *Reconstructing Schizophrenia*. London: Routledge.
Bentall, R.P. and Pilgrim, D. (1993) Thomas Szasz, crazy talk and the myth of mental illness. *British Journal of Medical Psychology* **66** (pt.1): 61–7.
Bifulco, A., Harris, T.O. and Brown, G.W. (1992) Mourning or inadequate care? Re-examining the relationship of maternal loss in childhood with adult depression and anxiety. *Development and Psychopathology* **4**: 119–28.
Blaxter, M. (1990) *Health and Lifestyles*. London: Routledge.
Borkovec, T.D. and Newman, M.G. (1998) Worry and generalised anxiety disorder. In A.S. Bellack and M. Hersen (eds) *Comprehensive Clinical Psychology: Volume 6*. London: Pergamon.
Bowlby, J. (1953) Some pathological processes set in train by early mother–child separation. *Journal of Mental Science* **99**, 265–72.
Bowlby, J. (1969) *Attachment*. London: Hogarth Press.
Boyle, M. (1991) *Schizophrenia: A Scientific Delusion*. London: Routledge.
Brayne, C. and Ames, D. (1988) The epidemiology of mental disorders in old age. In B. Gearing, M.L. Johnson and T. Heller (eds) *Mental Health Problems in Old Age*. Chichester: Wiley.
Briere, J. and Runtz, M. (1988) Post-sexual abuse trauma. In G.E. Wyatt and G.J. Powell (eds) *Lasting Effects of Child Sexual Abuse*. New York: Sage.
Brown, G.W. and Harris, T.O. (1978) *The Social Origins of Depression*. London: Tavistock.
Brown, G.W., Harris, T.O. and Hepworth, C. (1995) Loss, humiliation and entrapment among women developing depression: a patient and non-patient comparison. *Psychological Medicine* **25**: 7–21.
Browne, K., Davies, C. and Stratton, P. (eds) (1988) *Early Prediction and Prevention of Child Abuse*. London: Wiley.
Busfield, J. (1988) Mental illness as a social product or social construct: a contradiction in feminists' arguments? *Sociology of Health and Illness* **10**: 521–42.
Butzlaff, R.L. and Hooley, J.M. (1998) Expressed emotion and psychiatric relapse: A meta-analysis. *Archives of General Psychiatry* **55**: 547–52.
Cichetti, D., Toch, S.L. and Lynch, M. (1995) Bowlby's dream comes full circle: the application of attachment theory to role and psychopathology. *Advances in Child Clinical Psychology* **17**, 1–75.
Cole, M.G. and Bellavance, F. (1997) Depression in elderly inpatients: a meta-analysis of outcomes. *Canadian Medical Association Journal* **157**: 1055–60.
Copeland, J.R.M., Dewey, M.E., Wood, N., Searle, R., Davidson, I.A. and McWilliam, C. (1987) Range of mental illnesses amongst the elderly in the community: prevalence in Liverpool using AGECAT. *British Journal of Psychiatry* **150**: 815–23.

Coulter, J. (1973) *Approaches to Insanity*. New York: Wiley.

DH (2005) *Mental Capacity Act*. London: Department of Health.

Dimock, P.T. (1988) Adult males sexually abused as children; characteristics and implications for treatment. *Journal of Interpersonal Violence* 3: 203–21.

Dinos, S., Stevens, S., Serfaty, M. *et al.* (2004) Stigma: the feelings and experiences of 46 people with mental illness. Qualitative study. *British Journal of Psychiatry* 184: 176–81.

Dover, S. and McWilliam, C. (1992) Physical illness associated with depression in the elderly in community-based and hospital patients. *Psychiatric Bulletin* 16: 612–13.

Eastman, M. (1984) *Old Age Abuse*. Portsmouth: Grosvenor Press.

Erikson, E.H. (1998) *The Life Cycle Completed* London: Norton.

Fairbairn, W.R.D. (1952) *An Object-Relations Theory of the Personality*. New York: Basic Books.

Faulkner, A. and Layzell, S. (2000) *Strategies for Living. A Report of User-Led Research into People's Strategies for Living with Mental Distress*, London: Mental Health Foundation.

Gelder, M., Mayou, R. and Cowen, P. (2001) *Shorter Oxford Textbook of Psychiatry*. Oxford: Oxford University Press.

Gorbien, M.J., Bishop, J. and Beers, M.H. (1992) Iatrogenic illness in hospitalised elderly people. *Journal of American Geriatric Society* 40: 1031–47.

Gove, W.R. (1984) Gender differences in mental and physical illness: the effects of fixed roles and nurturant roles. *Social Science and Medicine* 19(2): 77–91.

Guze, S.B. (1989) Biological Psychiatry: Is there any other way? *Psychological Medicine* 19: 315–23.

Harlow, H.F. (1961) The development of affectional patterns in infant monkeys. In B.M. Foss (ed.) *Determinants of Infant Behaviour*. New York: Wiley.

Harlow, H.F. and Zimmerman, R.R. (1959) Affectional responses in the infant monkey. *Science* 130: 421.

Home Office (2000) *Domestic Violence: Revised Circular to the Police.*, HOC 19/2000. London: Home Office.

Hydle, I. (1993) Abuse and neglect of the elderly: a Nordic perspective. *Scandinavian Journal of Social Medicine* 2(2): 126–8.

Kay, D., Beamish, P. and Roth, M. (1964) Old age mental disorders in Newcastle upon Tyne: part 1, a study of prevalence. *British Journal of Psychiatry* 110: 146–8.

Kemker, S.S. and Khadivi, A. (1995) Psychiatric education: learning by assumption. In C.A. Ross and A. Pam (eds) *Pseudoscience in Biological Psychiatry: Blaming the Body*. New York: Wiley.

Kendler, K.S., Neale, M.C. and Kessler, R.C. (1992) Major depression and generalised anxiety disorder: some genes (partly) different environments? *Archives of General Psychiatry* 49, 109–116.

Kennedy, I. and Grubb, A. (1994) *Medical Law* (2nd edn). London: Butterworth.

Kirby, S.D., Hart, D.A., Cross, D. and Mitchell, G. (2004) *Mental Health Nursing: Competencies for Practice*. Basingstoke: Palgrave Macmillan.

Laing, R.D. and Esterson, A. (1964) *Sanity, Madness and the Family, Volume 1: Families of Schizophrenics*. London: Tavistock.

Lowenthal, M. (1965) Antecedents of isolation and mental illness in old age. *Archives of General Psychiatry* 12, 245–54.

Mann, A.H., Graham, N. and Ashby, D. (1984) Psychiatric illness in residential homes for the elderly: a survey in one London Borough. *Age and Ageing* 13: 257–65.

Marshall, J.R. (1990) The genetics of schizophrenia: axiom or hypothesis? In R.P. Bentall (ed) *Reconstructing Schizophrenia*. London: Routledge.

Maule, M., Milne, J. and Williamson, J. (1984) Mental illness and physical health in older people. *Age and Ageing* 13: 349–56.

Milligan, C., Gatrell, A. and Bingley, A. (2004) 'Cultivating health': therapeutic landscapes and older people in northern England. *Social Sciences and Medicine* 58: 1781–93.

Minett, R. with Members of the North East Warwickshire User Involvement Project. (2005) Partnership with the service user. In R. Tummey, *Planning Care in Mental Health Nursing*. Basingstoke: Palgrave Macmillan.

Moncrieff, J. and Crawford, M.J. (2001) British psychiatry in the 20th century: observations from a psychiatric journal. *Social Science and Medicine* **53**: 349–56.

Morris, R.G., Morris, L.W. and Britton, P.G. (1988) Factors affecting the emotional well-being of the care-givers of dementia sufferers. *British Journal of Psychiatry* **152**: 147–56.

Murphy, E. (1982) Social origins of depression in old age. *British Journal of Psychiatry* **141**: 135–42.

Murphy, E., Smith, R., Lindesay, J. and Slattery, J. (1988) Increased mortality in late life depression. *British Journal of Psychiatry* **152**: 347–53.

Nazroo, J.Y., Edwards, A.C. and Brown, G.W. (1998) Gender differences in the prevalence of depression: artifact, alternative disorders, biology or roles? *Sociology of Health and Illness* **20**(3): 3112–330.

Orbell, S., Hopkins, N. and Gillies, B. (1993) Measuring the impact of informal care. *Journal of Community and Applied Social Psychology* **3**: 149–63.

Pilgrim, D. and Rogers, A. (2005) The troubled relationship between psychiatry and sociology. *International Journal of Social Psychiatry* **51**(3), 228–41.

Post, F. (1969) The relationship to physical health of the affective illnesses in the elderly. *Proceedings of the Eighth International Congress of Gerontology*, Washington, DC.

Rank, O. (1929) *The Trauma of Birth*. London: Paul, Trench & Trubner.

Read, J., Agar, K., Argyle, N. and Aderhold, V. (2003) Sexual and physical abuse during childhood and adulthood as predictors of hallucinations, delusions and thought disorder. *Psychology and Psychotherapy: Research, Theory and Practice* **76**: 11–22.

Repper, J. and Perkins, R. (2003) *Social Inclusion and Recovery: a Model for Mental Health Practice*, London: Baillière Tindall.

Rhodes, A. and Goering, P. (1998) Gender differences in the use of outpatient mental health services. *Journal of Mental Health Administration* **21**(4): 338–46.

Sayce, L. (2000) *From Psychiatric Patient to Citizen: Overcoming Discrimination and Social Exclusion*. London: Macmillan.

Sanders, A.R., Detera-Wadleigh, S.D. and Gershon, E.S. (1999) Molecular genetics of mood disorders. In D.S. Charney, E.J. Nestler and B.S. Bunney, *Neurobiology of Mental Illness*. Oxford: Oxford University Press.

Scottish Government (2000) *Adults with Incapacity Act*. Edinburgh: Scottish Government.

Smith, R. (1987) *Unemployment and Health: A Disaster and a Challenge*, Oxford, Oxford University Press, cited in C.D. Mathers and D.J. Schofield (1998) The health consequences of unemployment: the evidence. *Medical Journal of Australia* **168**: 178–82.

Snowden, J. and Donnelly, N. (1986) A study of depression in nursing homes. *Journal of Psychiatric Research* **20**, 327–333.

Spagnoli, A., Foresti, G., MacDonald, A. and Williams, P. (1986) Dementia and depression in Italian geriatric institutions. *International Journal of Geriatric Psychiatry* **1**: 15–23.

Stakettee, G. S. and Frost, R.O. (1998) Obsessive compulsive disorder. In: A.S. Bellack and M. Hersen (eds) *Comprehensive Clinical Psychology: Volume 6*. London: Pergamon.

Stein, J., Golding, J., Seigel, J. *et al.* (1988) Long term psychological sequelae of child sexual abuse: the Los Angeles epidemiologic catchment area study. In: G.E. Wyatt and G.J. Powell (eds) *Lasting Effects of Child Sexual Abuse*. New York: Sage.

Szasz, T. (1992) *A Lexicon of Lunacy: Metaphoric Malady, Moral Responsibility and Psychiatry*. New Brunswick: Transaction.

Tien, A.Y. (1991) Distribution of hallucinations in the population. *Social Psychiatry and Psychiatric Epidemiology* **26**: 287–92.

Tummey, F. (2003) Domestic abuse: the hidden factor, *Mental Health Nursing Journal* **23**(2): 4–6.

Tummey, R. and Smojkis, M. (2005) Primary mental health care. In: R. Tummey, *Planning Care in Mental Health Nursing*. Basingstoke: Palgrave Macmillan.

van Os, J., Hanssen, M., Bijl, R.V. and Ravelli, A. (2000) Strauss (2000) revisited: a psychosis continuum in the normal population. *Schizophrenia Research* **45**: 11–20.

Wade, T.J. and Cairney, J. (1997) Age and depression in nationally representative sample of Canadians. *Canadian Journal of Public Health* **88**, 297–302.

Whitfield, C., Dube, S., Felitti, V. and Anda, R. (2005) Adverse childhood experiences and hallucinations. *Child Abuse and Neglect* **29**: 797–81.

Widiger, T.A. and Trull, J.T. (1994) Personality disorders and violence. In J. Monahan and H.J. Steadman (eds) *Violence and Mental Disorder*. Chicago: Chicago University Press.

Winnicott, D.W. (1958) *Collected Works*. London: Hogarth Press.

Winnicott, D.W. (1967) The location of cultural experience. *International Journal of Psychoanalysis* **48**, 370–8.

8

Iatrogenic Abuse

Robert Tummey and Francesca Tummey

BRIEF CHAPTER OUTLINE

This chapter discusses abuse within mental health services. Although the subject is somewhat contentious, it is addressed with firm conviction. Iatrogenic influences are first detailed to form a frame of reference. Then three distinct sections are identified as the main points of debate. To commence, the influence of the mental health service environment is explored, including ward, hospital and philosophy. This leads into the impact of mental health treatment and abuse experienced through medication, mental health laws, the use of force and the flawed concept of insight. Then the text moves to explore the 'difficult to face' area of individual clinician abuse. Attitude completes this section, followed by a discussion on current improvements and future vision.

Introduction

The American Iatrogenic Association (2002) states that 'iatrogenic' refers to the harmful consequences of actions by physicians and other health professionals; from the Greek *Iatros*, 'physician', and *-genic*, 'induced by'. This chapter will specifically explore harmful consequences or abuse within mental health care.

Abuse occurs in mental health care against the people served, through the staff, the systems, the care, the emphasis and the power. It may not be the purpose and it may be 'dressed' in a way that can be justified, but it does occur in the care delivered every day. The nature of such discussion can be a disturbing reminder of human depravity and capability. It also serves as stark evidence that 'care' does not always afford people protection or asylum, but can create and re-create the chilling experiences of abusive relationships that harm and deprive.

Abuse is a term that means many things to many different people. It is an ever-present feature of human life through the paradox of human struggle and triumph. Being abused can create a victim or, indeed, an inspiration from victim to victor (Coleman and Smith, 1997). Abuse can be maliciously intended by the persecutor, or an unintentional experience. It is a widespread phenomenon that transcends boundaries of culture, social class, gender and sexuality. The term includes sexual and physical violence perpetrated against another person, as well as emotional abuse or neglect that promotes power, control and dominance over another. All aspects can influence the mental health of the person or result from the mental health issues a person has.

Psychodynamic theory suggests that unresolved dynamics of childhood experience can be re-created within an adult dynamic. A health professional might contribute to re-creating the unresolved dynamics of a service user's childhood experience. An example would be rejection. If the service user has been repeatedly rejected by those in significant attachment positions in childhood they may unconsciously re-create the dynamics of rejection with all carers/caregivers in adulthood. This aspect is what Berne (1964) termed a 'life script' that can be played out time and again. All too often, the counter-transference from these dynamics encourages abuse from the carer/caregiver. For all mental health professionals, awareness of abusive dynamics should be paramount.

In current mental health care there are a number of things to celebrate. Many services are providing, at least, adequate or above adequate support and involve service users in their treatment. Collaboration is expected, and for many it is now a reality. Exploring such areas is a worthy pursuit. However, for the purpose of this chapter, a critical view is required to expand the story and examine situations – overt or covert, meant or unintentional – where abuse of the service user may occur. This is not intended to cancel out the good work being achieved, but a reminder of influences and attitudes that undermine good work.

The chapter therefore examines the nature of such abuse and the kind of experiences that can have a profound effect on the user of mental health services. It will take into account the various guises abuse takes on within mental health care, from the impact of the service environment, the treatments offered in the name of science and the individual clinician's influence. It will be an exploration of where the prevalence lies and how abuse is experienced from within the culture of the mental health system. Each section will detail the iatrogenic influences that impact on service users, past and present. A discussion and future vision will tie the aspects together in an attempt to look to the future through a reduction in the unintentional blind adherence or intentional power dynamic that is endemic in the mental health system.

Iatrogenic influences

According to the World Health Organization, abuse is broken down into four categories: neglect, emotional, sexual and physical. So how do these abuses manifest themselves in the mental health system? Here is a brief overview, with further detail explored later in the chapter.

Neglect: The 'disliked service user' being avoided and ignored; the person deemed 'attention-seeking' receiving no compassion; the complainant being treated with contempt; the office nurse not interacting with service users; the omission of a clinical procedure; service-focused care; engagement in counter-transference.

Emotional: Staff teasing service users in front of others or when alone; being on constant alert as an in-patient; a lack of decisions being made by clinicians; a lack of decision-making power; use of a language of power/jargon; giving messages late from carers/callers, service users not being listened to.

Sexual: The exposure of others (intentional or unintentional); disinhibited service users; vulnerable young people (particularly women); the defenceless; use of mixed wards that house the abused with abusers; predators; service users' sexuality being dismissed; a lack of privacy.

Physical: The use of force (verbal, numbers of staff, holding, restraint, seclusion); medication (poly-pharmacy) and possible side effects; poor environment, omission of GP input or treatment, lack of physical care, substandard physical examination and equipment.

Mental health care is often at the frontline of providing for people who are displaced, disturbed or abused. Services stretch across the age range and attempt to consider gender, social and cultural influences within their own circumstances and experience. The multi-disciplinary team (MDT), consisting of professionals who specialize in mental health care, work together on the premise that they provide a service for the benefit of the service user. Care teams discuss risk assessment and will take abuse into account (whether the person has been abused or is an abuser), generally focusing on risk to self or others. Rarely would iatrogenic risk be considered, involving overt or covert abuse from the actual care provided and the mental health system. Protocols may be adhered to, but the impact of care or control of the individual will fall second to the immediacy of protecting the person and the public. This, itself, can be an abuse.

In the mental health system, abuse has been perpetuated for many years (Barnes and Bowl, 2001) through the same persecution, which targeted witches, Jews, gypsies and homosexuals (Szasz, 1974). This has taken various forms, including abuse of power, the overuse of medication, use of restraint, seclusion and so on. All can be justified within a system that is unsure whether to look after the person in distress or lock them up (Laurance, 2003); care for the person or control them (Barnes and Bowl, 2001). Most abusive interactions can be attributed to the service user's attitude and behaviour. However, what of the carer or caregiver, whether relative or health professional? There is a definite reality that service users can be caught in a dynamic that escalates situations that are familiar to their experience and which favour the staff becoming abusive, coercive and controlling.

Iatrogenic abuse within mental health service environment

Mental health care throughout the ages has been brutal, with chaining and whipping until the eighteenth century. Then, even with the new-found liberalism of the nineteenth and twentieth centuries, through attempts to tolerate behaviour the environment of asylums was abusive and harsh, with little care. These abusive surroundings offered frightening sounds, poor diet, bland hospital garb, the dead hand of routine, the bludgeoning of individuality, and so on and so on (Shorter, 1997). The sound of keys and locked doors, the noise of distress, the air of unpredictable tension prevailed.

Even today the environment takes its toll on service users and staff alike. As Chamberlain (1988: 5) so powerfully states, 'I spent five months as a patient in six mental hospitals. The experience totally demoralised me ... after hospitalisation, I was convinced of my own worthlessness.' There are abusers beside the abused in mental hospitals and the drug-fuelled perpetrators of social misery. An acute in-patient care unit is a frightening place for anyone to have to stay, not least to receive care and have time to improve from distress. Often the places are grim, degrading, broken and hostile. Rarely are they homely, inviting and bright. Hospitals can also seem more like warehouses for the sedation of the utterly victimized and powerless (Johnstone, 2001).

Indeed, in Laurance's book *Pure Madness* (2003), Jan Wallcraft, a mental health researcher, talks of a service user who committed suicide for fear of coercion and acknowledged powerlessness. She says: 'She needed a helper who would respect her for the person she really was, rather than seeing her as a helpless victim of delusions who needed to be artificially numbed into forgetfulness.' Once in hospital, one would hope that service users receive some form of solace and recuperation. However, they can be drugged and held until some of their circumstances alter at home or their observed behaviour changes. This observation can be achieved in several ways, including direct knowledge of their whereabouts and checks at various times.

The actual use of CCTV and night-time observation has been introduced in a UK ward. This highlights control versus therapeutic engagement and caring. Page and Meikeljohn (2004) found that the literature highlights the fact that observations are often a service user-controlling experience born out of fear of litigation. On their ward, the service user can make the choice between CCTV or traditional methods of observation. Page and Meikeljohn considered the ethical concerns and claim that there are few barriers. Also, they suggest that, in their experience, traditional observation providing opportunity for interaction is more theoretical than practical. However, this takes away the human element and the possibility of 'being with' a person during their distress. The use of technology in mental health care has not been embraced, say the authors. This is interesting, as the human element appears to be missing from their position, taking a grim look into the possible future of withdrawing attention and watching from afar. How depressing.

Then there is identification in the community. To find the ward or community centre is not too difficult. In order to identify their actual position, usually great big 'lunatic' signs point the way. They may say, *Mental* Health Unit, *Mental* Health Centre, *Psychiatric* Unit, Centre for *Psychiatry*, Community *Mental* Health. This can be useful to establish where to go for an appointment, but also alerts everyone else as to the purpose of the visit. This can be stigmatizing and perpetuate discrimination among the community. Generally people fear the mentally ill, and highlighting them is not a benefit. Surely alternatives could be explored.

The homes in which people with mental illness are expected to live are often substandard and inappropriate to their needs. People with mental illness generally come from lower socioeconomic backgrounds or cascade to this status. They are more likely to be unemployed or in low-income employment and therefore live in lower socioeconomic environments, with poor housing and lack of protection. Housing estates have gangs, neighbours from hell, children poking fun, harassment, exploitation and so on. High-rise flats pose a danger in terms of suicide risk, as they make residents feel isolated and penned-in, and their height leads to fatality for those who jump. Housing policy has since changed to reflect concern. The Supporting People Programme across the UK (DCLG, 2003; Scottish Government, 2005) ensures that vulnerable people are housed appropriately. Now, where possible, people diagnosed with schizophrenia will not be housed above ground level or in any high-rise building. This applies to those people seeking rehousing and not those in situ.

Approach

With the case for different approaches and emphasis in mental health service provision, division is apparent and hostility clear. This comes about through rivalry, competition for funding and the fight for resources. In the debate over early intervention, a recent article attempted to provide opposing positions. This does not develop awareness of services but appears quite damaging. The service user is seemingly lost to the argument for further power and the possibility of the clinician being right.

On one hand, Anthony Pelosi (a psychiatrist) believes early intervention teams are an abuse of resources and service users. He argues that for every service user appropriately treated during a prodromal phase of schizophrenia there are many more, with similar clinical features, who will never develop this uncommon illness. He believes vulnerable service users will receive powerful antipsychotic medications unnecessarily and equally, powerful and potentially dangerous psychotherapy. Also, it is not aimed at the middle-aged or elderly and will be used only during an arbitrary 'critical period'. Max Birchwood (a psychologist) disagrees and states that early intervention is a way forward, as current care is based on late intervention that has a low intensity and haphazard and coercive intervention (Pelosi and Birchwood 2003). Healthy debate is good, but who is right?

Iatrogenic abuse from mental health treatment

Various treatments and approaches are available in mental health care, but none are as dominant as the biomedical model. The biomedical bias of psychiatry is apparent for various reasons, as described by Rogers and Pilgrim:

1. It medicalizes psychological distress.

2. It improves the medical status of psychiatry.

3. It is perpetrated by the profit-making drug companies (major tranquillizers and medications for all ills, including the side effects generated).

4. It is cheaper to deliver than talking therapies.

5. Physical/biomedical treatments can be imposed in the absence of co-operation.

6. The behavioural impact of psychotropic drugs provides a spurious illusion that bio-determinism has been proven (Rogers and Pilgrim, 2005: 144). As Szasz (1985) suggests, 'since Theocracy is the rule of God or its priests, and democracy the rule of the people or of the majority, pharmacracy is therefore the rule of medicine and of doctors'.

Each aspect above raises the concern for the extreme position of power afforded psychiatry and the ability to perpetuate abusive relationships with the people they serve. All prescribed psychotropic medications given to service users have side effects. Their use can be poorly managed or monitored, and although improvements of one aspect of life can be evident, it is often at the expense of other areas. Sedation is also a concern. Service users are reduced to a more manageable stupor with flattening of affect. Indeed, this can become a daily facet of their life. In hospital, pro re nata (PRN) is additional prescribed medication to be given as required at the discretion of the nurse and provides further opportunity to sedate and suppress through additional antipsychotic medication or benzodiazepines. This then becomes the 'mad signature' of a person with the mental illness, reduced to a dribbling, dull, blunted individual who shuffles through the ward, corridor or community; controlled by the drug. This has led us from the previously accepted social construction of illness to the now replaced corporate (drug company) construction of disease (Moynihan, Heath and Henry, 2002).

In 2001 approximately 43 million prescriptions of antipsychotics were issued in France, Germany, Spain, Italy, the UK and the USA (IMS, 2003). There is evidence of increased use in older adults and younger people (whether they have psychosis or not). Interestingly, there is little evidence they even treat any illness but, instead, numb the senses and responses to stimuli. Indeed, the preponderance of evidence shows that continual medication therapy for all service users with schizophrenia does more harm than good, even increasing the likelihood that a person will become chronically ill (Whitaker, 2004). This has not improved under the atypical antipsychotic revolution. The superiority afforded atypicals is questionable (Ross and Read, 2004). Atypicals do have an improved side-effect profile, but still produce significant reactions with no increased benefit (see Ross and Read, 2004). The most common is weight gain and all the increased physical health problems associated with increased weight. Conventional antipsychotics have a more severe side-effect profile than atypicals, with the most extreme being neuroleptic malignant syndrome. This occurs in between 0.2 per cent and 1.9 per cent of individuals treated with antipsychotics. In spite of all the evidence that antipsychotic medication is harmful in long-term use and would be better used in a selective manner, psychiatry is moving in the opposite direction and prescribing to an even larger patient population (Whitaker, 2004).

Other treatments include the use of electroconvulsive therapy (ECT). The NICE (2003) guidance recommends limiting its use for certain conditions and reads as a cautious view of the procedure. There may be cases of success, but essentially it cannot be said to be effective, with anterograde and retrograde memory loss and memory dysfunction very real consequences (Read, 2004b). ECT is the passing of sufficient electricity through a human brain to cause a *grand mal* seizure. This can be administered through a unilateral or bilateral approach, that is, either passing the electric current through one side or both sides of the brain. In addition to the frightening nature of the treatment, ECT recipients also experience a complex range of emotional responses, including feelings of humiliation, increased compliance, failure, worthlessness, betrayal, lack of confidence and degradation and a sense of having been abused and assaulted (Johnstone, 1999).

The treatment given to service users is not always overt medical prescription, but also includes the very damaging message it conveys. When mental illness is considered deviant behaviour the message is negative. Rogers and Pilgrim (2005) explored the work of Goffman, who describes the negotiation of deviance as the 'betrayal funnel' and the 'degradation ritual'. The betrayal funnel is a conspiratorial relationship between relatives of patients forcibly admitted to hospital and the receiving professionals – participating in the process of civilian to patient status, thus converting protest into illness and placing into asylums those who otherwise would be challenging the established order (Shorter, 1997). The degradation ritual is the removal by professionals of a person's everyday identity and the stripping of their usual sense of self (Goffman, 1967). This is demoralizing.

Strauss makes a direct link between negative messages that people are given and their 'demoralization'. Some treatment efforts may inadvertently create the opposite effect intended. People with schizophrenia are often told they have a disease, all their lives, that involves major functional impairment and a lifelong need for medication. Withdrawal, isolation, apathy and anhedonia are partly a manifestation of demoralization. Many of what are described as negative symptoms are attributable to demoralization (Strauss, 1985). This is further compounded by the fact that the very construct of schizophrenia, as employed by clinicians and researchers all over the world, remains disjunctive and therefore scientifically meaningless (Read, 2004a).

Use of force

Any use of force or *restraint* of an individual for whatever purpose and for whatever outcome can result in a misuse of staff and an infringement of the service user's rights. It is a rather primitive response and takes a number of people to perform. Indeed, it takes a number of people who are all at the same practical skill level to carry out a successful restraint that minimizes harm to the service user and staff. Often this is sadly lacking and the staff are all at varying degrees of competence and also confidence. This breeds fear and mistakes. It could be questioned by each person in the team, but unfortunately takes place due to the rush of adrenaline and fulfilling some meaningless obligation to stick to consequences discussed with the service user. All or some may secretly harbour concerns and wish the whole experience did not happen. Exerting power over another human being has a cost. Indeed, to replicate their experience of *powerlessness* and retraumatizing them further away from trust is immeasurable. This is what occurs.

In the UK *seclusion rooms* and the process of secluding a person were seemingly outlawed during a period of fresh hope and false expectation. Seclusion was viewed as the *punishment* it is. To protect staff, people were restrained, escorted away and forced into an enclosed space, often surrounded by the grunting and shouting of a gang of staff. One minute, taking a person's liberty for non-compliance of medication, violent behaviour or being plain crazy and unmanageable was the order of the day the next minute, suddenly it wasn't. Some time in the 1990s it became unspeakable to seclude someone and seclusion rooms quickly became decommissioned. Now seclusion rooms have returned, as they are viewed as a better way to manage a person in distress than using restraint for long periods, with possibly fatal consequences (for further information see the David 'Rocky' Bennett Inquiry; Blofeld *et al.*, 2003).

Insight: the danger of knowledge, or lack of it

Further disempowerment of the person suffering from mental illness is assured through the intriguing concept of insight. If they do not believe they have schizophrenia then their insight is impaired ... Indeed, they must be mad! This is rather a mixed bag of interesting clinical decision-making and ostensibly, understanding how the disadvantaged service user perceives him or herself. The issue appears to be whether the service user agrees with the clinician or not. If they do not, then they have 'no insight'. There is very little or no concern for the service user's understanding of the experience.

Research will show that there are links between poor insight and poor outcomes in schizophrenia. Goldberg *et al.*'s (2001) research supports a relationship between ratings of poor insight and a psychotic diagnosis, increased psychiatric symptoms, poorer social skills and negative medication attitudes. Is this not obvious? In further research, there is evidence to support the hypothesis that insight is related to the psychopathology of schizophrenia. People with schizophrenia, wherever they are, vary in their willingness to accept an illness attribution of their state. They are more likely to do so if they are anxious (Saravanan *et al.*, 2007). So, does this mean that experiences can be accepted by the person as a cultural, spiritual or emotional process, but that they can only be accepted as illness if the person is consumed by fear?

Although a causal chain connecting poor insight with poor adherence to treatment and poorer outcome is straightforward, numerous studies provide differing results. The association with long-term adherence remains unclear – problems relating to definition and study designs are considered responsible for inconclusive findings (Lincoln, Lullmann and Rieff, 2007). This also occurs for the very subject of schizophrenia (Leo and Joseph, 2002; Read, 2004a). Could this be due to the subjective concept of insight, applied to further justify coercion and treatment?

A lack of insight is not used to cloak the very real concern for a high proportion of people diagnosed with schizophrenia, namely, the risk of suicide. This does not make headlines, whereas homicide does. As a result of raised concern from the public via the media, the switch from care to containment has taken place (Laurance, 2003). Once labelled 'schizophrenic', a person cannot object to or resist treatment – that would be evidence of their mental disorder. Branded as a mental patient, he or she is no longer a credible witness, even about his or her own mind. A medical record is therefore just like a criminal record, with one difference: the person can never clear his or her name (Laurance, 2003).

Iatrogenic abuse from individual clinicians

Creating a distance between self and service user can be apparent through the concept of *othering*. This attitude creates dependence and aligns to a superior difference over the inferior 'service user'. As Keen (2003) states, it includes the type of language and tone used and the use of jargon; being unclear, indirect, invalidating and non-collaborative; imposing rules; and thinking, however unconsciously, that people with schizophrenia are childlike, dangerous and incomprehensible. These 'us and them' distinctions underpin prejudice and discrimination and pervade mental health services. People with mental health problems are devalued and so those who work with them, by association, are also devalued (Repper and Perkins, 2003). To preserve status it can be tempting for staff to dissociate from devalued service users and amplify difference. The 'othering' or 'us and them' concept requires exposing and challenging.

There can be *overt expressions* of anger by staff through being callous, unkind and even violent towards service users, as described in the brave New Zealand Confidential Forum (see DIA, 2007). Also, members of staff sometimes need to get their own way through power, influence, status, height, language and so on. *Covert expressions* of communication also produce equally abusive dynamics. Poor or dismissive interaction with service users can be demeaning. This may extend to using others to convey messages and manipulating the person or situation through the use of power, by exploiting position in the team. Having a *low expectation* that the person *will* be abusive or uncooperative can be a problematic perception that perpetuates a negative stance from staff and leaves the person labelled and undermined.

A *lack of resources* is often cited as an issue through low staffing ratios in both inpatient and community. This can lead to abuse and a culture of cruelty through neglect and unsafe practice (Coppock and Hopton, 2000). Indeed, if the members of staff have *poor standards/skills* then this exacerbates the opportunity for mistakes and bad practice. The impaired use or lack of therapeutic skill determines poor management of the person and any risk factors. It is then increasingly difficult to practise in safety. Other aspects can be the misuse of the Mental Health Act (1983) and Mental Health (Care and Treatment) (Scotland) Act (2003), with compliance used as an excuse to assert power over an individual.

Dynamics between staff can be a damaging influence and evoke tensions. Coming from a different values-base can present a dilemma of *discipline, envy and ignorance*. Seeing something different in the situation aids progress or hinders the process, depending how it is viewed. Negative staff dynamics create a rivalry akin to siblings and can produce a 'turf war'. Each discipline should be contributing to effective management, communicating concern and raising debate that fosters the best outcome for the service user. However, who should be responsible for provision of the key assessment? Is collaboration of effective change a given? Are clinicians pieces of a larger multidisciplinary team jigsaw, with a valued resource and knowledge base? Some *barriers* include professional disputes over ownership of psychological distress (Barnes and Bowl, 2001); defending one's own turf, clarity of role and wastage of scarce resources (Carnwell and Buchanan, 2005); alongside a lack of interdisciplinary understanding, professional ignorance, arrogance or fear and a concern for shared involvement. The individual service user is then lost in the process of disputes, while the clinician is safe in the protected fold of their discipline.

The abusive clinician can be hidden by the very services that purport to care, as their aim is to 'first do no harm'. If an individual health professional is abusive, there should be procedures accessible to the service user for swift scrutiny of practice. Where there is a blurring of accountability, a new organization has emerged to meet the need. WITNESS is the only charity in the UK exclusively concerned with breaches of trust in professional relationships. It supports survivors of abuse at the hands of psychotherapists, psychiatrists, counsellors, psychologists and other health and social care professionals. Their stance is inclusive and states that abuse is when the therapist has betrayed the client's trust. (For more information on WITNESS please refer to www.popan. org.uk). A recent study has shown that often abuse is perpetrated by male practitioners in senior positions, in their 50s and 60s. Statistics show that men make up 60 per cent, women, 21 per cent and the rest are gender unknown (Pointon, 2002).

Attitude

There exists a wide divergence between the interests of psychiatry and service users. If the purpose of the system is to meet service user needs, then the system is irrational, with an iatrogenic dysfunction and organizational weakness (McCubbin and Cohen, 1996). This may be apparent to all involved, but rarely challenged. The attitude that prevails is apathy at best and superiority at worst. This considerable imbalance of power sits in favour of the professionals and is linked to the abuse of service users with mental illness, with assertive or knowledgeable users being seen as threatening (Minett *et al.*, 2005), or even considered as part of their pathology and attributed to a personality disorder.

Abuse and discrimination are not just restricted to the mental health system but also occur in the primary care sector (Kumar, 2000). When mental health services were converting to community care, the hospitals were shutting and many service users were discharged to fend for themselves. Often they were ignored or inadequately housed and lacked appropriate support from Primary Health Care. In fact, some had no access to a General Practitioner (GP). Public fear can also be health professionals' fear. Some GPs would be reluctant to take on people with a diagnosis of mental illness; therefore the person's mental and physical health would suffer further as a result of alienation from services.

Discussion and future vision

There are many reasons why abuse is part of mental health services. From the environment, treatment and attitude, abuse is present and should be challenged. In mental health service terms, there may never be a world without abuse. The presence of abuse alerts us to the human experience. From despair comes change, hope and advocacy of others. Being abused can be a victorious platform that provides strength. There are positive changes already taking place. *User movements* have grown over recent years to develop the voice of the consumer. These are not confined to mental health, with patient power exerted in various departments and specialties in physical care. The expert patient is a growing phenomenon in cancer care and many other longer-term conditions. They provide support, self-help groups and an avenue for consulting and sharing information. Other aspects of *user involvement* are speaking up for others, offering protection to service users and providing staff training on user experience. Many user organizations have emerged to offer service-user advocacy and advice through to user movements and forums.

A *no-blame culture* for staff is now apparent. Clinicians are able to come forward if they inadvertently abuse or witness another member of staff's abuse. This leads to *increased reporting* of incidents, helping to establish what is occurring and at what level. This entail informs the *audit process* which is taking place across many services. Medical information and service-user notes are being reviewed for the purpose of professional and ethical treatment, plans and outcomes measuring up to expectations. *Professional accountability* embodies the integrity and professional reputation of each discipline. Each discipline has their own code of conduct or ethics that informs the judicial process and provides a more transparent complaints procedure for service users. Indeed, many health professionals can be named and shamed by their governing body if found guilty of an offence against a service user. Full details of the circumstances of the offence are listed, alongside the process of investigation and outcome of the hearing.

There are a number of factors required by mental health professionals to avoid and eradicate abuse in mental health services. An overview is considered below.

Society – there should be a change in attitude towards people with mental illness and an expectation of care provision and protection, and a person's rights must be observed and monitored. Within society, people are experiencing abuse and abusing, giving rise to negative consequences for the victims and ultimately, for society itself. There are also positive aspects to all this, such as attempts to reduce or eradicate unacceptable behaviours. A brief, less than exhaustive list might include:

- *zero tolerance* of any antisocial behaviour

- *heightened awareness* in communities and neighbourhoods

- *political correctness* of language and discrimination

- *human rights* agenda within Europe and across the world

- *expectation* of people

- *self-help groups* encouraged and supported by statutory agencies

- *information explosion* and increased access to data.

Each of these aspects is an example of life in a society that is more educated, knowledgeable and assertive. This has influence on the people who live and work within that society and includes mental health professionals and those using mental health services.

Service – zero tolerance of abuse is apparent. Ethical standards are in place and adhered to. With sufficient resources, adequate care could be achieved. In order to achieve such professional intervention, *effective line management* is essential. This will enable protection from the ongoing pressures in higher management. Also, it will provide direct knowledge and support that allows the professional to perform their role autonomously, but with guidance. To assist in the process of people work, *collegial support* provides grounding and open access to others in the same line of work. This provides the opportunity to discuss, offload and advise, which is invaluable to the clinician. For a more formalized process, establishing *clinical supervision* is an essential means of gaining understanding of the barriers that may hinder progress with a client or amplify the clinical aspects that work. One of the remaining facets of working within mental health care as a professional should be the desire and intention of ensuring service-user benefit.

Service clinician – attitude, supervision, effective communication sharing and having a common goal are important. The health professional from each discipline should have a professional protocol that ensures service users are not subject to abuse within the service or directly from the clinician. It is expected that this would include overt or covert abuse and indeed, purposeful, deliberate or accidental abuse. For mental health professionals, prerequisite standards should prevail. These will include areas like *appropriate training and education* recognized by a governing body and set against national standards. This would lead to *relevant qualifications* that are current and endorsed by the governing body. An *appropriate level of knowledge* will then be attained that can be used to the benefit of the clientele served. When engaging with the service user or group, the professional should employ a necessary and applicable *skill set for interventions* such as therapeutic engagement, communication, de-escalation and restraint.

Service user – important here are the complaint process, support groups to voice concerns and information gaining and sharing. A number of factors should be considered for improvement of collaboration with service users, including:

- Mental health services have had a poor record of collaboration with service users. Partnership is a worthwhile aspiration, but co-operation should increase first (Bassett, 2000).

- Pro-choice in services for people to determine what and whom they would prefer should be advocated. This includes the opportunity to request a specific gender (although this can also be questioned), a specific or similar culture within reason and the right to have an interpreter for using their own language to express their distress.

- Improved education and information access for all service users is a necessity.

- Evidence-based interventions reflecting clinical research should be offered.

- A skilled workforce will deliver such interventions through effective protocols and guidelines for provision.

Mental health interest groups do not command political power proportional to the numbers affected (Kelly, 2006). Support is necessary to provide a vision that will lift the dark veil of abuse, another taboo subject rarely discussed, which is uncomfortable and stirs emotion in people.

Conclusion

There are reasons, justifications and rules to abide by in any society and community. However, sometimes abuse can hide behind the norm or traditional practice of 'what has always been done'. If you have always done something in a certain way , then it must be wrong, because theory evolves and life and practices change. Things change and views differ as time goes by and may not reflect the view of the past or indeed, vision for the future. We have moved a long way from mechanical restraint, deep insulin treatment and ice baths, all performed in the name of treatment. Anything done in the service user's best interests needs to be fully justified.

The aim of this chapter has not been to point fingers or raise the temper of those working hard to provide a worthwhile service. It has not been any intention to deliver a negative chapter that highlights the 'ills' of mental health care. Rather, it is an attempt to provide a debate and probably a warning of what can go wrong, with awareness opening channels to prospective change. Abuse is abuse is abuse. It is not enough to explain it away or hide behind tradition, standards, policy or jargon.

EDITORS' QUESTIONS

Issues of difference

- How can gender-specific abuse be avoided in acute mental health care?
- In what way is iatrogenic risk age-related?
- How should the team avoid neglect of a service user's cultural needs?

Relevance to practice

- How do mental health professionals deal with concerns for a service user who is not responding to treatment in your service?
- In what ways can psychiatry reduce the iatrogenic risk of abuse in mental health care?
- How does each discipline contribute to the empowerment of the service user?

Investigate

- How is iatrogenic risk assessed in your service or practice?
- You discover a service user is not being heard. Consider how you respond as a health professional within your role.
- What contribution can you make to reduce iatrogenic impact?

Suggested further reading

Read, J.; Mosher, L. and Bentall, R. (eds) (2004) *Models of Madness: Psychological, Social and Biological Approaches to Schizophrenia*. Hove: Brunner-Routledge.
Repper, J. and Perkins, R. (2003) *Social Inclusion and Recovery: A Model for Mental Health Practice*. Baillière Tindall.

References

American Iatrogenic Association. (2002). www.iatrogenic.org/ [accessed 29/01/08].
Barnes, M. and Bowl, R. (2001) *Taking over the Asylum: Empowerment and Mental Health*. Basingstoke: Palgrave Macmillan.

Bassett, T. (2000) Is partnership possible? *Open Mind* **104**: 12–13.

Berne, E. (1964). *Games People Play: The Basic Handbook of Transactional Analysis*. New York: Ballantine Books.

Blofeld, J. *et al.* (2003) *Independent Inquiry into the Death of David Bennett*. Cambridge: Norfolk, Suffolk and Cambridgeshire Strategic Health Authority.

Carnwell, R. and Buchanan, J. (2005) Learning from partnerships: themes and issues. In *Effective Practice in Health and Social Care: A Partnership Approach*. Maidenhead: Open University Press.

Chamberlain, J. (1988) *On our own*. London: MIND. In M. Barnes and R. Bowl, *Taking over the Asylum: Empowerment and Mental Health*. Basingstoke: Palgrave Macmillan, 2001.

Coleman, R. and Smith, M. (1997) *Victim to Victor 1: Working with Voices*. Runcorn: Handsell.

Coppock, V. and Hopton, J. (2000) *Critical Perspectives on Mental Health*. London: Routledge.

DCLG (2003) *Supporting People Programme*. Department for Communities and Local Government. www.spkweb.org.uk/ [accessed 29/01/08].

DIA (2007) *Te Aiotanga: Report of the Confidential Forum for Former In-Patients of Psychiatric Hospitals*. Wellington, New Zealand: Department of Internal Affairs.

Goffman, E. (1967) *Interaction Ritual*. Harmondsworth: Penguin.

Goldberg, R.W., Green-Paden, L.D., Lehman, A.F. and Gold, J.M. (2001) Correlates of insight in serious mental illness. *Journal of Nervous and Mental Disorder* **189**(3): 137–45.

IMS (2003). http://www.imshealth.com [accessed 4/09/07].

Johnstone, L. (1999) Psychological trauma after ECT. *The Survivor* **16**: 32–5.

Johnstone, L. (2001) Psychiatry, still disagreeing. *Clinical Psychology* **7**: 28–31.

Keen, T. (2003) The person with schizophrenia. In P. Barker (ed.), *Psychiatric and Mental Health Nursing: The Craft of Caring*. London: Arnold.

Kelly, B.D. (2006) The power gap: freedom, power and mental illness. *Social Science and Medicine* **63**(8): 2118–28.

Kumar, S. (2000) Client empowerment in psychiatry and the professional abuse of clients: where do we stand? *International Journal of Psychiatry in Medicine* **30**(1): 61–70.

Laurance, J. (2003) *Pure Madness: How Fear Drives the Mental Health System*. London: Routledge.

Leo, J. and Joseph, J. (2002) Schizophrenia: medical students are taught it's all in the genes, but are they hearing the whole story? *Ethical Human Sciences and Services* **4**: 17–30.

Lincoln, T.M., Lullmann, E. and Rief, W. (2007) Correlates and long-term consequences of poor insight in patients with schizophrenia: a systematic review, *Schizophrenia Bulletin*. Schizophrenia Bulletin Advance Access published online February 8, 2007 [accessed 23/08/07].

McCubbin, M. and Cohen, D. (1996) Extremely unbalanced: interest divergence and power disparities between clients and psychiatry. *International Journal of Law and Psychiatry* **19**(1): 1–25.

Mental Health Act (1983) Department of Health, London: Stationery Office.

Mental Health (Care and Treatment) (Scotland) Act (2003) Edinburgh: Scottish Government.

Minett, R. *et al.* (2005) Partnership with the service user. In R. Tummey, *Planning Care in Mental Health Nursing*. Basingstoke: Palgrave Macmillan.

Moynihan, R., Heath, I. and Henry, D. (2002) Selling sickness: the pharmaceutical industry and disease mongering. *British Medical Journal* **324**: 886–90.

NICE (2003) *Guidance on the Use of Electroconvulsive Therapy*. London: National Institute for Clinical Excellence.

Page, M. and Meikeljohn, C. (2004) CCTV and night-time observations. *Mental Health Practice* **7**(10): 12–15.

Pelosi, A. and Birchwood, M. (2003) Is early intervention for psychosis a waste of valuable resources? *British Journal of Psychiatry* **182**: 196–98.

Pointon, C. (2002) Protecting the client. *Counselling and Psychotherapy Journal* **13**(9): 12–16.

Read, J. (2004a) Does schizophrenia exist? In J. Read, L. Mosher and R. Bentall (eds) *Models of Madness: Psychological, Social and Biological Approaches to Schizophrenia.* Hove: Brunner-Routledge.

Read, J. (2004b) Electroconvulsive therapy. In J. Read, L. Mosher. and R. Bentall (eds) *Models of Madness: Psychological, Social and Biological Approaches to Schizophrenia.* Hove: Brunner-Routledge.

Repper, J. and Perkins, R. (2003) *Social Inclusion and Recovery: A Model for Mental Health Practice.* Baillière Tindall.

Rogers, A. and Pilgrim, D. (2005) *A Sociology of Mental Health and Illness* (3rd edn). Milton Keynes: Open University Press.

Ross, C.A. and Read, J. (2004) Antipsychotic medication: myths and facts. In J. Read, L. Mosher and R. Bentall (eds) *Models of Madness: Psychological, Social and Biological Approaches to Schizophrenia.* Hove: Brunner-Routledge.

Saravanan, B., Jacob, K.S., Johnson, S., Prince, M., Bhugra, D. and David, A.S. (2007) Assessing insight in schizophrenia: East meets West. *British Journal of Psychiatry* 190: 243–9.

Scottish Government (2005) *Homes for Scotland's People: A Scottish Housing Policy Statement.* www.scotland.gov.uk/Publications/2005/03/20793/53989 [accessed: 29/01/08].

Shorter, E. (1997) *A History of Psychiatry: From the Era of Asylum to the Age of Prozac.* Chichester: John Wiley.

Strauss, J.S. (1985) Negative symptoms: future developments of the concept. *Schizophrenia Bulletin* 11: 3.

Szasz, T.S. (1974) *The Myth of Mental Illness: Foundations of a Theory of Personal Conduct* (rev edn). New York: Harper & Row.

Szasz, T.S. (1985) *Ceremonial Chemistry: The Ritual Persecution of Drugs, Addicts, and Pushers.* Holmes Beach, FL: Learning Publications.

Whitaker, R. (2004) The case against antipsychotic drugs: a 50-year record of doing more harm than good. *Medical Hypotheses* 62: 5–13.

WITNESS: Against abuse by health and care workers. www.popan.org.uk [accessed 29/01/08].

9

Psychological Trauma

Derek P. Farrell

BRIEF CHAPTER OUTLINE

Within this chapter, a critical look at psychological trauma will first explore the multifaceted context of human trauma. Through the use of statistics and case examples the text brings the subject to life. The history and discourse of trauma then allows the author the opportunity to outline the journey taken and how individuals react to war, terrorism and tragedy. The reader is then given some of the evidence for how information is processed and what traumatic memory entails. This section also includes the diagnostic criteria for the presentation of post-traumatic stress disorder (PTSD). A discussion of litigation then follows to determine the influence of the legal system and insurance companies on the victims of PTSD. Future directions of psychological trauma conclude the chapter.

Introduction

When studying psychological trauma, three distinct characteristics emerge in considering humans. First, that our vulnerability to trauma is not just a physical manifestation, but is also a profoundly psychological phenomenon that can cause duress long after physical healing has taken place. The second is that as humans we possess an unnerving ability to inflict hurt, harm, and in some cases immense evil. We are reminded both of our powerfulness – for example in the case of warfare – and our powerlessness – in relation to tsunamis, earthquakes and other natural disasters. Thirdly, we possess an innate potential to heal, a propensity to survive, and in some cases to 'psychologically grow' in the aftermath of traumatic events. Martin Luther King (1965) captures all three characteristics in this succinct quote: 'We shall have to repent in this generation, not merely for the hateful words and actions of the bad people, but for the appalling silence of the good people.' Each of these three aspects of humanity is essential in considering psycho-traumatology.

The term 'trauma' comes from the ancient Greek word meaning 'to wound' or 'to pierce'. The context in which it was first used was in reference to soldiers who had suffered injury resulting from the piercing of armour; and that somehow the soldiers' defences, designed to protect them from death, had been exposed and then overpowered (Spiers and Harrington, 2001). This sense of the physical defences being 'overwhelmed' provides a useful parallel when considering our current understanding of psychological trauma. Since our existence on this planet our world has been dramatically affected by an array of traumas, either by design or default, by force of nature, by human endeavour, by act of God, or of human failing. Perhaps the most remarkable consideration therefore is that no matter how large or small the trauma has been, the human race continues to survive. It survives for better or worse, for richer or poorer, but survives nonetheless, indicating our strength, tenacity, resilience, salvation, hope and potential.

Many of the world's religions contain large swathes of violence and aggression, of pain and suffering, within their history. The Bible itself makes many references to cruelty, abuse and inhuman treatment, including child sacrifice, infanticide, rape, incest and prostitution, with the New Testament recounting the emergence of Christianity following on from the barbaric torture and crucifixion of Jesus of Nazareth. Following the atrocities of the two world wars of the twentieth century, an abundance of institutions became established in the aftermath of these traumas, such as the United Nations, the World Health Organization, the European Court of Human Rights, and there were many developments in human rights legislation. All these sprang up in recognition of the pain and suffering that went before them, fuelled by the belief that in learning from our past we can offer a better future for future generations.

The United States has played a paradoxical part in enhancing our understanding of psychological trauma. On 11 September 2001 over 3000 people lost their lives when two planes crashed into the Twin Towers in New York. This act resulted in a dramatic shift in world order, leading to subsequent invasions of Afghanistan and Iraq. The death of 3000 people is unquestionably a devastating event and of major political significance. However, there is a different perspective. In the United States the total number of road deaths for 2001 was 42,169 (OECD, 2006). In 1990 road traffic accidents were the ninth highest leading cause of death worldwide. It is estimated that by 2020 this will have risen to the third highest (Dyrerov and Raundlen, 2005).

Road crashes can affect anyone, but young road users suffer the heaviest burden from road traffic injuries, whether from tragic early death or from long-term disability that may affect the rest of their lives. In Europe, road traffic injuries are the main cause of death for children and young people aged between 5 and 24, wiping out over 30,000 lives a year (WHO, 2007). Road traffic crashes are the leading cause of death among young people aged between 10 and 24, according to a new WHO report. The report, *Youth and Road Safety*, says that nearly 400,000 young people under the age of 25 are killed in road traffic crashes every year, and millions more are injured or disabled.

One of the many consequences of the horrendous aftermath of the Vietnam War was the devastating effect the conflict had on countless men and women in the military services. What was perplexing about this syndrome was not only an individual's exposure to the sheer horror of war, but that such a traumatic experience resulted in a fundamental personality change and a significant alteration of that person's level of functioning. In many ways this syndrome is effectively a product of its social time, and is quintessentially a post-Vietnam War North American conceptual framework. A point to consider is that had the affected soldiers returned as 'heroes' to a nation with overwhelming community and social support, an effective and inclusive health-care system, and a system of compensation, things might have been very different (Williams, 2006).

Horowitz's (1975) important paper on the phenomenology of traumatic reaction, published in the *Archives of General Psychiatry*, played a significant part in influencing the American Psychiatric Association in the notion that the traumatized individual was assailed by intrusive and emotionally disturbing memories which are physiologically arousing. This disturbance causes the individual to use avoidant strategies to ward off these distressing thoughts, feelings and images. The *Diagnostic and Statistics Manual of Mental Disorders* (APA, 1980) accounted for this syndrome as that of post-traumatic stress disorder (PTSD). It was determined that PTSD had three core features: intrusive recollections, avoidant behaviour and increased physiological arousal. This new conceptual framework was a defining aspect within the field of psycho-traumatology and certainly paved the way in terms of generating innovative psychological treatment methods and interventions. In turn this generated a strong empirical understanding of trauma characteristics.

However, it could be argued that the United States has also contributed to creating a world order that, by its very nature, induces psychological trauma, effectively a country that fulfils the roles of perpetrator, healer and victim. The date of 11 September was a defining moment in North American history in creating a nation unquestionably traumatized by its experience while endeavouring to establish its own healing and resolution. In the post 9/11 era more American soldiers have lost their lives in the Iraq conflict than who died in the collapse of the Twin Towers (World News, 2007).

In 2006 the Israeli government sanctioned a war on Lebanon where over 3,600 people were killed. What was poignant about this conflict as portrayed by the world's media was that the distinction between that of 'perpetrator' and 'victim' was being defined by a matter of perspective; often these highly emotive and powerful words were considered ambiguous and interchangeable, defined either by the individual, group, culture, religion, politics, gender, economics, etc., with a morally neutral perspective being an anathema.

A characterological perspective of trauma reveals that it is indeed a multifaceted phenomenon; the main catalysts of trauma being that of war, conflict, terrorism, sexual abuse, domestic violence and natural disasters. Part of its character is that it is complex, disturbing, constantly changing and at times contradictory:

- Since the Second World War there have been approximately 145 conflicts throughout the world, of which the United States has been involved in over 56 (Blum, 2007).

- Concerns about terrorism have also grown exponentially since 11 September 2001.

- Growth in communications technology enables people to be traumatized from the safety of their own homes on a previously unprecedented level.

- Between 1993 and 2003, 2 million children were killed and 6 million children injured or permanently disabled in war zones throughout the world.

- Of war-exposed survivors, one million children have been orphaned and 20 million displaced to refugee camps.

- In conflicts civilians comprise 80–90 per cent of all those who die or are injured, with most of the casualties being children and their mothers (Barenbaum, Ruchkin and Schwab-Stone, 2004).

- Rape is a more common problem than war; more women are raped than men go to war (Fortune, 1995).

- Around the world at least one woman in every three has been beaten, coerced into sex or otherwise abused in her lifetime, with most abusers being a member of her own family (Heise, Ellsberg and Gottemoeller, 1999).

- In the United States the health-related costs of rape, physical assault, stalking and murder committed by an intimate partner exceed $5.8 billion each year (Centre for Disease Control and Prevention, 2003).

- General population surveys suggest that between 13 and 30 per cent of individuals have been exposed to one or more natural disasters in their lifetime (Green and Solomon, 1995).

- In 1993 there were 53,000 deaths from 261 natural disasters, and in 2003, 83,000 deaths from 337 natural disasters (International Strategy for Disaster Reduction, 2004).

- In the USA approximately 80 people are killed each day by firearms.

- In 2006 1,591 people were executed by their own governments, the main offenders being China, Iran, Pakistan, Iraq, Sudan and the United States.

- By the end of 2006 the Iraqi government reported that since the invasion of 2003 over 12 000 national police officers have been killed.

An argument exists, therefore, that the domain of psychological trauma is increasingly a messy, complicated, and at times counter-productive, protracted business, which is rapidly developing into a huge industry taking on a life of its own. This is exemplified by the case of a motorcyclist, a 32-year-old man called Ray. Ray was involved in a serious motor vehicle accident through a side-impact collision with a car. The driver had gone through a red light and was later certified as being 'well over' the alcohol limit. Ray experienced horrific injuries. Later, in hospital, it was deemed that the surgical removal of his right leg was essential. Ray's life was never the same again.

After five years of complex litigation Ray was eventually awarded £950,000 in compensation. However there are several pertinent and intriguing factors in Ray's story in relation to psychological trauma. Many of the issues Ray found the most disturbing related to events that took place after the index trauma. Following completion of the litigation and compensation process, Ray's legal bill came to over £80,000. Ray was significantly distressed that his lawyers economically benefited from the lengthy process of litigation that he considered had been 'self-sustained'. In many ways Ray was emphasizing an important point in that the protracted element of proceedings has a secondary gain for legal representatives, while potentially compounding problems for the clients. Furthermore, through this five-year period he was subjected to a great many medico-legal assessments regarding his physical care, rehabilitation, prosthetics, phantom limb pain and psychiatric, psychological, economic, social and occupational welfare, with Ray recounting that many of these assessments were hostile, confrontational, contradictory and protracted. He was diagnosed with 'severe PTSD' by one clinician, and by another as a 'malingerer'. When he eventually received his compensation he was overwhelmed by the dramatic insurgence in the number of 'new' friends he suddenly acquired, many of whom made requests for money, perceiving him now to be 'extremely rich'. His best friend said, 'I'd lose my leg for that amount of money.'

As a consequence of the actions of one drink driver, Ray lost his leg, his job, his marriage, his way of life and many of his hobbies. Ray's story is not unique. However, it does tell us that losing his leg was extremely traumatic and devastating, but in exploring the totality of his trauma experiences, so was much of the 'help and support' that he received in the aftermath. The police report on the accident declared, 'there was absolutely nothing *Ray* could have done to have prevented the accident'.

The history and discourse of trauma

In the last 200 years the discourse of psychological trauma has constantly altered and adapted as our understanding of the phenomenon becomes more enriched and enlightened through a greater acquisition of knowledge. This discourse has proved sometimes productive, sometimes pejorative, sometimes insightful and sometimes provocative. But as the language has altered over the course of time, psychological trauma has a long history.

It is not unusual for ancient knowledge to be lost only to be rediscovered many centuries later. That some people display a number of physiological and psychological symptoms in the aftermath of war, disasters and traumatic experiences has been known for nearly three millennia. The earliest references to psychological trauma appear from the Greco-Trojan wars in approximately 1500 BC. Spiers and Harrington (2001) submit that the story of trauma is one of enlightenment and forgetfulness. It is an account of knowledge gained and lost time and time again, a history characterized by criticism and denial. Even now there are those who question the legitimacy of PTSD, people who view it purely as a late twentieth-century, western phenomenon, a product of a victim and compensation culture and weakness of character. Kardiner and Spiegel (1947) were of the view that each investigator who undertakes to study these conditions considers it his or her sacred obligation to start from scratch and work at the problem as if no one had ever done anything about it before. Following the Great Fire of London in 1666 Samuel Pepys, the English diarist, recounted hyper-arousal, disturbed sleep, nightmares, feelings of detachment, increased irritability and a loss of interest in his usual activities. Professor Leo Ettinger, a psychiatrist who studied survivors of Nazi concentration camps, and himself an Auschwitz survivor, declared:

> War and victims are something the community wants to forget; a veil of oblivion is drawn over everything that is painful and unpleasant. We find the two sides face to face; on one side is the victim who perhaps wishes to forget but cannot, and on the other all those with strong often-unconscious motives who intensely wish to forget and succeed in doing so. The contrast is painful to both sides. The weakest one remains the losing party in this silent and unequal dialogue.
>
> (Ettinger, 1980, quoted in Herman, 2001: 8)

In the conflict between that of the victim and perpetrator it is arguably morally impossible to remain neutral. Such conflict, by its very nature, generates an affect, often a powerful emotional response. The consequence of this lack of neutrality is a corollary effect; bystanders are ostensibly forced, either by design or default, to take sides. Bera (1993) offers an example of this after studying the response of church congregations following the disclosure that its pastor had allegedly committed a sexual misdemeanour. What Bera discovered was that when congregations are presented with this situation, they fracture, with the congregation caught in the polarity between pastor and victim. What is striking within this phenomenon is often the lack of balance. The more powerful dynamic prevails in that it is often very tempting to take the side of the perpetrator rather than the victim. All the perpetrator wants is for the bystander to say nothing, appealing to the universal desire to see, hear and speak no evil. The victim, on the contrary, wants the bystander to share the burden of the pain. The victim requires action, engagement and remembering. In order to escape accountability the perpetrator does everything to promote forgetting; secrecy and silence are the perpetrator's first line of defence. If secrecy fails, then the perpetrator attacks the credibility of the victim. If the victim cannot be silenced, then the perpetrator ensures that no one will listen. To this end the perpetrator will portray an impressive range of arguments, from the most banal denial to the most sophisticated and elegant rationalization; it never happened, the victim lies, the victim exaggerates, the victim brought it on themselves, it is time to forget the past and move on. A perpetrator's argument often proves irresistible when the bystander faces them in isolation. Without a supportive environment the bystander usually succumbs to temptation to look the other way (Herman, 2001). A tragic paradox of trauma is that one of its primary casualties is that of truth itself.

> I was first on the scene after the bomb went off. There was just carnage everywhere. It was a mess. I didn't join the police force for this. But I knew my job was to hold the line and not let anybody through. As I stood there, I couldn't breathe, I felt as if my chest was about to explode. I desperately wanted a drink of water. Then I saw the Chief Inspector coming towards me. He took one look at the scene, and then he glared at me, and promptly rollicked me for not wearing my tie properly, telling me that I was a disgrace to the RUC. There were dead people all around, but all I can remember is being reprimanded for undoing my tie. When we got back to the station, nobody talked about it. My sergeant gave me a bottle of whiskey and told me to go home. I think that was my debriefing. Every day I see those images, every day I feel those same feelings of being scared, of thinking I am going to die. Next time it will be me. I can't bear that train station, even today. I hate it. That station is death.
>
> (statement from Joseph, ex-Royal Ulster
> Constabulary (RUC) police officer, 2003)

The above transcript is from a statement relating to a significant terrorist incident which occurred on 4 December 1971 when the Protestant Ulster Volunteer Force (UVF) exploded a bomb in a Catholic area of Belfast, Northern Ireland, which killed 15 civilians and caused widespread damage and destruction. Some thirty years later Joseph continues to be significantly affected by the events of that day back in 1971, soon after which he left the force, and spent the next many years trying to find resolution through the use of alcohol, with the consequences of marital breakdown, financial hardship and social disintegration. It was only 32 years later that he eventually sought help and found that he was certainly not alone in what he was experiencing, but what was more important was that his symptoms made sense. But the question is, in what way?

There are a number of distinct elements to Joseph's story:

- reliving – constant flashbacks and intrusive recollections of what had happened, including frequent nightmares

- hyper-arousal – feeling constantly anxious, hyper-vigilant, and having an exaggerated startle response

- emotional dysregulation – having difficulty expressing his feelings and emotions, disengaging him from his social contacts

- avoidant behaviour – he avoids certain places and is reluctant to get close to people for fear of losing them.

In order to take into account the myriad of symptoms people encounter in response to a trauma, responses just like Joseph's, researchers have suggested post-traumatic stress disorder, or PTSD (APA, 1980, 1995, 2000), as the diagnosis that best suits the syndrome commonly seen in survivors (Bisson and Andrew, 2007; Brewin and Holmes, 2003; Foa, Keane and Friedman, 2000; van der Kolk *et al.*, 2007; Yule, 2000). This disorder presumes that the person has experienced a traumatic event that involved actual or threatened death or injury to either themselves or others, where they felt fear, helplessness or horror. However, the very label itself implies that it is the nature of the event that is traumatic. In DSM-III-R (APA, 1980) it considered the trauma as 'an event outside the range of usual human experience'. This presented a problem in that the focus centred upon the stressor rather than the way in which an individual made sense, or in some cases did not make sense, of that stressor. Examples being that two people may experience the same stressor yet respond to that stressor in a completely different way. When 96 Liverpool football fans lost their lives at Hillsborough stadium, Sheffield in 1989, there were over 40,000 people in the ground that day, yet not all of them developed PTSD. The DSM-IV Criterion (309.81; APA, 1995) is clearer in relation to this; however, although Criterion A acknowledges the importance of objectivity there also needs to be cognisance of the way in which an individual interprets these events.

There are three symptom clusters which, within the updated *Diagnostic and Statistical Manual of Mental Disorders* (DSM-IV-TR; APA, 2000: 309.81), state that classification for PTSD requires the survivor to be in 'clinically significant distress or impairment in social, occupational, or other important areas of functioning'. The main symptom clusters, or effectively the essential hallmarks of PTSD, are intrusion, such as flashbacks or nightmares where the traumatic experience is re-experienced; avoidance, where the person tries to reduce exposure to people or things that may bring on re-experiencing the phenomenon; and finally hyper-arousal, which are all physiological indicators of increased anxiety. What the PTSD framework ostensibly enables is that its intrinsic elements be considered within the context of a syndrome with core aetiology, rather than just a list or catalogue of symptoms.

Wilson and Keane (2004) provide an interesting and encompassing dimension of PTSD from a psychobiological perspective in six categories that represent the epigenesis of PTSD: traumatic event(s), psychobiological substrates, organismic processes, symptom development, PTSD clusters and adaptive behavioural configurations. Wilson and Keane consider that the organismic processes in PTSD are manifestations of synergistic interactions between both biological and psychological systems. The biological aspects are neurophysiological in that they are innate and pre-programmed, whereas the psychological involves perception, memory, cognition, learning, personality processes and the self-structure.

However, according to Ehlers and Clarke (2000), a number of the above effects may be generated by cognitive distortions and maladaptive beliefs about the self and the interpersonal world that become part of a person's cognitive schemata when the trauma occurred. Jehu, Klassen and Gazan (1986) and Kennerley (1996) both indicate that the pathogenic effects of negative core beliefs associated with a trauma such as sexual abuse, for example, pose a significant component of post-trauma reactions. The cognitive effects of negative self-evaluation, guilt, helplessness, hopelessness and profound distrust may act as contributory factors in producing the affective and interpersonal problems that can often cause so much distress and difficulty for survivors (Briere, 1996; Donaldson and Gardner, 1985; Farrell, 2003; McCann and Pearlman, 1990).

In considering these cognitive components further there are two pertinent cognitive components, that of assimilation and accommodation; which have been proposed as key factors in the interpretation of trauma (Ehlers and Clarke, 2000; McCann, Sakheim and Abrahamson, 1988; Resick and Schnicke, 1990; Smucker et al., 1995). In the first instance trauma experiences actually defy assimilation, existing instead as dissociated material that re-emerges as flashbacks, nightmares, flashes of affect or memory fragments (Horowitz, 1976). The information itself may be altered in order to be assimilated into already existing schemas. With accommodation, however, the existing schema is altered in order to take in discrepant information (Hollon and Garber, 1988). As Smucker (2004) affirms that a child's schema related to self-efficacy may become disrupted to the point that a schema of powerlessness becomes more dominant, trust may be replaced by mistrust, and a schema of self as positive may be distorted so that a sense of the self as stigmatized and evil is formed. Because child sexual abuse is by definition pathological, it is not therefore surprising that changes in existing schemas are predominantly pathogenic. Several basic themes emerge in the thinking of adult abuse survivors that suggest the influence of maladaptive schemas. The presence of degrading self-perceptions may indicate that fundamental assumptions about the benevolence and meaningfulness of the world, self-worth and personal invulnerability become distorted by the trauma of the sexual abuse, and that maladaptive schema formation occurs (Janoff-Bulman, 1985, 1992; Young, 1990).

The proportion of people exposed to traumatic events who then go on to develop PTSD varies according to the nature and severity of the event. According to NICE (2005), the probability of developing PTSD after a traumatic event is 8–13 per cent for men and 20–30 per cent for women. This translates to an annual prevalence rate in the UK of between 1.5–3 per cent, so a Primary Care Trust with a population of 170,000 will have an estimated 2,500–5,000 people with PTSD, which within a doctor's general practice of 5,000 patients would amount to approximately 75–150 people. A differing context is that in the aftermath of the Pakistan earthquake in October 2005, where over 73,000 died, the prevalence of PTSD in the surviving population was approximately 51 per cent (Montazeri and Baradaran, 2005). However, generally ascertaining the percentage of people who suffer PTSD after experiencing a trauma is not easy. One of the major reasons for this is that in many studies of disasters the PTSD criterion has not been used (Hodgkinson and Stewart, 1991). In a study by Loughrey et al. (1988), of those affected by terrorist bombings, 23 per cent had symptoms of PTSD, while in assessment of survivors of the Zeebrugge ferry disaster, for compensation purposes, 90 per cent were considered to be suffering from PTSD (Williams and Yule, 1988).

There are three important determinants in ascertaining the likelihood of developing PTSD, namely (a) the severity of the trauma (e.g., violence, fear of death); (b) whether injuries were sustained; and (c) multiple traumatization

(Resick and Schnicke 1990, 1993). When all three risk factors have been present, PTSD is much more likely in the vast majority of cases (Kilpatrick, Veronen and Resick, 1982). Interestingly, Mayou, Bryant and Duthie (1993), in a study on the psychiatric consequences of road traffic accidents, showed that PTSD symptomatology was strongly associated with horrific memories of the accident. However, they found that the syndrome did not occur in any subject who had been unconscious or amnesic from the accident. O'Brien and Nutt (1998) stipulate that loss of consciousness leads to an absence of any memory of the incident, therefore the patient will have no horrific memories, flashbacks or nightmares and consequently will not re-experience the incident repeatedly. This may prevent the progressive activation of other brain circuits that together form the brain substrate for PTSD, the consequences being that the lack of memory means that there is less reason to avoid the relevant cues to the event, with the probable result of less avoidance behaviour. However, this may be true of certain single traumas, but it has a decreased significance in cases of multiple trauma. People subjected to prolonged, repeated trauma develop an insidious progressive form of PTSD that invades and erodes the personality. While the victim of a single acute trauma may feel after the event that she or he is 'not themselves', the victim of chronic or multiple trauma may feel changed irrevocably, or may even lose the sense that they have any self at all (Herman 2001). PTSD tends to also be more severe and longer-lasting when the traumatic event is of human design, for example sexual abuse, torture, terrorist attacks or war atrocities, rather than natural disasters, earthquakes, tsunamis, floods, hurricanes and so on.

Trauma affects a whole range of core psychological functions. These include regulation of feelings; thinking clearly about what happened in the past and was currently happening; ways in which feelings are expressed by the body; and people's views of themselves, strangers and intimates. Van der Kolk (1996) considers that the older the victim, the shorter the duration of the trauma, and the more likely it is for the person to develop only the core PTSD symptoms; the longer the trauma, and the less protection, the more pervasive the damage. What is interesting about O'Brien and Nutt's (1998) observations are that despite requiring further empirical evidence, loss of consciousness would appear to protect the person from PTSD, probably by preventing the encoding of traumatic memories. This process of encoding is an important phenomenon within the PTSD syndrome.

One of the most significant developments in PTSD research has been that of neuroimaging. Scientists have gained a huge advantage from being able to see how a brain malfunctions. This has provided insights in to how the brain stores and recalls memories. Pierre Janet (1989 [1899]) was the first researcher to clearly articulate the difference between ordinary and traumatic memories. One of the early pioneers of brain imaging with PTSD was Bessel van der Kolk. In an attempt to elucidate neurobiological underpinnings of PTSD, subjects with PTSD underwent positron emission tomography (PET) images of the brain. Under conditions of extreme stress there is a failure of hippocampal memory-processing with the consequence that this impairs the ability to integrate incoming sensory data into a coherent autobiographical narrative. This means, therefore, that the remaining sensory elements are 'unintegrated and unattached'. Or as van der Kolk *et al.* (2007) succinctly declare, in cases of trauma the thalamus doesn't work properly.

In people with PTSD the brain's ability to process the traumatic event becomes impaired. This traumatic memory is stored in the part of the brain known as the amygdala, which is responsible for the evaluation of emotional meaning of incoming stimuli. It is thought that the amygdala helps integrate internal representation of the external world. One of the important aspects of this is the survival instinct; the hippocampus triggers the 'fight, flight or fright' response when something dangerous occurs. There are three brain regions, connected by neural pathways that are critically important in regulating fear-related behaviours. The first is the pre-frontal cortex, which participates in assessing danger. The second is the amygdala, which is a major constituent of the emotion-producing limbic system. The third is the hypothalamus. In response to signals from the pre-frontal cortex, amygdala and hippocampus, the hypothalamus directs the release of hormones that support motor responses to perceived threats. In terms of PTSD our pre-frontal cortex knows that it is the present and that the individual is not in present danger; however the amygdala, the emotional memory, has been triggered in such a way that it considers that the event is happening all over again. PTSD is effectively a breakdown in communication between the pre-frontal cortex and the amygdala.

Yet trauma is not just a collection of symptoms conceptualized under the auspices of PTSD. These symptoms are an outward indicator of an individual's response to such a traumatic event. Prior to the trauma the individual is a person with a history and sense of identity. The trauma shatters the assumptive world of that individual with sometimes devastating consequences. The individual's invulnerability has gone; the world is now seen as darker, maligned, evil, chaotic, and unpredictable or even dangerous place.

Information processing and traumatic memory

As mentioned previously, one of the most influential models of PTSD is Horowitz's (1986a, 1986b) contribution of information processing, which combines both psychodynamic and cognitivist theories. It purports that traumatic experiences disrupt an individual's life by producing a block in both cognitive and emotional processing (Bracken, 2002; Shapiro, 1989, 1995; Young, 1995). When a traumatic event occurs this presents information which conflicts with pre-existing schemas, and thus an incongruity arises which in turn gives rise to stress. This provokes a stress response that involves a reappraisal of the event and a revision of these schemas. Shapiro (1989, 1995, 2001), van der Kolk (1996), van der Kolk, Boyd and Krystal (1985), van der Kolk *et al.* (2007) and van der Kolk and van der Hart (1995) all purport that when someone experiences a severe psychological trauma, it appears that an imbalance may occur in the nervous system, caused perhaps by changes in neurotransmitters such as adrenaline. This imbalance results in the system of information processing then being unable to function and that the information acquired at the time of the event, including images, sounds, affect and physical sensation, is maintained neurologically in its disturbing state.

The original material which is held in this distressing, excitatory state-specific form continues to be triggered by a variety of internal and external stimuli and is expressed in the form of nightmares, flashbacks and intrusive recollections. The disturbing aspects of these dysfunctionally stored memories result in the information stored being manifested by all elements of the trauma, including intrusive symptoms, negative assimilation and physiological affect. The characteristics of this negative assimilation are that these pervasive thoughts are there, and are self-referencing, illogical and generalizable.

In order to remember new information it is necessary to have prior knowledge about the subject; while one-trial learning exists, most skills and knowledge are acquired by repetition (Brandsford and Johnson, 1972; Sherry and Schacter, 1987). Van der Kolk and van der Hart (1995) propose that people who possess a prior store of information about a particular area of knowledge tend to integrate new data related to that subject more easily than do people who have little or no prior knowledge, and thus assert that memory is an active and constructive process and that remembering depends upon existing mental schemas. Therefore this argument purports that new experiences can only be understood in the light of previous schemas, and that they are affected by particular internal and external conditions prevailing at the time. In fact Janet (1989 [1898]) observed that events are much more likely to be determined as traumatic when a person is tired, ill or under stress. The brain then organizes this sensory information into what Young (1987) defines as 'message patterns'. Yet in 1898 Janet commented:

> The person must not only know how to do it, but must also know how to associate the happening with the other events of his life, how to put it in its place in that life history which each one of us is perpetually building up and which for each of us is an essential element of our personality. A situation has not been successfully liquidated, has not been fully assimilated until we have achieved, not merely through our movements, but also an inward reaction through the words we address to ourselves, through the organisation of the recital of the event to others and to ourselves, and through the putting of this recital in its place as one of the chapters in our personal history.
>
> (1989 [1898], 25, 2:273)

What makes this so relevant to PTSD and in particular the significant shift between the DSM-III and DSM-IV diagnostic criteria is directly in relation to this issue of individual assimilation and accommodation of the traumatic experience, as such traumatic memories become fixed in the mind and are not altered by the passage of time or the intervention of subsequent experiences. These memories are repeated without modification (van der Kolk *et al.*, 1985).

In research with traumatized children and adults, van der Kolk and van der Hart (1995) suggest that in contrast to narrative memory, traumatic memories lack verbal narrative and context. According to Bruner and Postmand (1949) and Piaget (1973), a child's earliest memories are encoded in the sensory motor system, while visual representation becomes dominant between the ages of 2 and 7. By contrast, linguistic representation develops more slowly, and may not be fully integrated with the kinaesthetic and visual modes of representation until adolescence. These trauma memories are state-dependent in that the memories are reactivated when a person is exposed to a situation, or is in a somatic state reminiscent of the one during which the original memory was stored. These are then encoded in the form of vivid sensations and images, regardless of the victim's age, and cannot be accessed by linguistic means alone. In fact Beck and Freeman (1990) state that simply talking about the traumatic event may give intellectual insight about why a patient has a negative self-image, but it does not actually change the image. In order to modify the image, it is necessary to go back in time, as it were, and re-create the situation, as only then can cognitive restructuring occur.

Another important characteristic of trauma memories is that they can be unavailable for retrieval under ordinary conditions, tending to be 'fixed' in their original form and unaltered by the passage of time or subsequent experience.

Many traumatized people experience long periods in which they live in two different worlds: the realm of the trauma and the realm of their current ordinary life. Very often survivors struggle to reconcile these two coexisting worlds. Langer (1991) and Herman (2001) both agree that for some this duality may be permanent by not being able to shift the trauma memories into a narrative. In Langer's (1991) research into the oral testimonies of Holocaust survivors he recounts:

Witnesses are both willing and reluctant to proceed with the chronology; they frequently hesitate because they know that their most complicated recollections are unrelated to time. Trauma stops the chronological clock and fixes the moment permanently in memory immune to the vicissitudes of time. The unfolding story brings relief, while the unfolding plot induces pain (1991, 174–5).

Litigation and PTSD

There is also an economic problem in respect to PTSD relating to the notion of adversary. There are two parallel adversarial systems in relation to trauma. The first rests between that of the alleged victim and alleged perpetrator, and the second rests between both the legal system and insurance companies or compensation bodies. Survivors, in their search for justice, frequently recount evidence of re-traumatization as a consequence of this adversarial interplay, with an all too familiar outcome of justice not prevailing. This is compounded by the fact that there have been no changes to the legal system in relation to PTSD. However, the central question is still whether the person is really suffering as a direct result of the trauma, and the extent to which their life has been altered as a consequence.

Should the person be entitled to care and respect, or deserving of contempt, whether they are genuinely suffering or malingering, whether their histories are true or false, whether imagined or maliciously fabricated (Spiers and Harrington 2001)?

For survivors of trauma there are distinct advantages in seeking litigation. Often it is seen as a means of emancipation, where justice can be achieved through clearly defining appropriate responsibility and accountability. Many survivors acknowledge the importance of their stories being heard and believed, and that this can be extremely empowering, freeing people from the secrecy that often enshrouds their traumatic experience. With a guilty verdict there is potential vindication for the survivor as the attribution of blame and responsibility is shifted to the perpetrator. This can have a huge therapeutic value in that the credibility of the perpetrator is significantly affected, with the corollary of reducing risk for the future and a reduction in further victims. Litigation can offer psychological closure for survivors by challenging the pervasive secrecy that often enshrouds trauma.

Nonetheless, there are many disadvantages to pursuing litigation. In the vast majority of trauma cases litigation is often an extremely protracted process, lasting for several years. This, by its very nature, stifles emancipation as it fundamentally links the survivor back to the trauma events, creating many of the following characteristics:

- Stifled emancipation
- Connection with others
- Not obtaining closure
- Challenges credibility of victim
- Requires confrontation with abuser
- Procedural time lapse
- Litigation process itself
- Justice may not happen

- Over-responsibility
- Ethical dilemmas
- Metamorphosis of guilt and shame
- Disempowerment
- Media intrusion
- Negative impact of family and social support

Justice is expensive. Outcome is massively dependent upon a whole host of variables of which victim survivors have very little control and influence. The victim's voice is not as powerful as a self-sustaining industry where lawyers are often handsomely rewarded for the undertaking of the duty of care, yet often the consequences of survivors is of great significance. Much more infrequently do victim survivors find the judicial process healing and cathartic; many find it traumatic, devastating, counter-productive and retraumatizing.

An important development in response to litigation is that of restorative justice. Restorative justice, forgiveness and reconciliation are increasingly being considered as a replacement for more traditional, hard-line approaches to the types of wrongdoing that are especially psychologically damaging. However, clinical research as to the psychological benefits of these approaches is severely lacking.

Future directions of psychological trauma

At the present time the diagnostic classification guidelines for DSM-V are being considered. The likelihood is that the core aetiological framework for PTSD, namely intrusivity, hyper-arousal and avoidance, will remain the same.

However, there needs to be a refinement of the criteria for Section A. Presently it is too vague and needs to be narrowed down.

There is every indication that PTSD will increasingly become a more politicized diagnosis. The recent $660 million settlement by the Roman Catholic Archdiocese of Los Angeles to over 500 alleged victims of sexual abuse by members of the clergy bears testimony to that (Flaccus 2007). When such vast sums of money are involved, politics will feature as a dynamic.

However, there is a strong indication that the future for PTSD research will be in the direction of neuroplasticity, the ability of the brain to effectively rewire itself by allowing neurons in the brain to compensate for injury and to make adjustments in response to new situations or to changes in the environment. Developing a better understanding of brain functioning is a vital part of the equation in furthering knowledge about PTSD. The more difficult challenge is to work towards not creating victims in the first place. The question is; can such a utopia exist? The answer rests in our hands.

EDITORS' QUESTIONS

Issues of difference

▩ In what ways can a psychological trauma have an impact on sexuality?

▩ How is trauma linked to child abuse, and what are the long-term effects?

▩ How is a natural disaster perceived in different cultures?

Relevance to practice

▩ How do mental health professionals assess previous trauma?

▩ An adult service user discloses childhood sexual abuse from their past. How do you respond as a health professional within your role?

▩ How does each discipline contribute to the effective treatment and care of a person suffering PTSD following a road traffic accident?

Investigate

▩ What are the recent advancements in PTSD research?

▩ How is psychological trauma dealt with in your service or practice?

▩ How does the process of litigation hinder the possible psychological progress of the person suffering from a traumatic event?

Suggested further reading

Bracken, P.J. (2002) *Trauma: Culture, Meaning and Philosophy*. London: Whurr.
Herman, J.L. (2001) *Trauma and Recovery*. New York: Harper Collins.

References

APA (1980) *Diagnostic and Statistical Manual of Mental Disorders III.* Washington, DC: American Psychiatric Association.

APA (1995) *Diagnostic and Statistical Manual of Mental Disorders IV.* Washington, DC: American Psychiatric Association.

APA (2000) *Diagnostic and Statistical Manual of Mental Disorders IV TR.* Washington, DC: American Psychiatric Association.

Barenbaum, J., Ruchkin, V. and Schwab-Stone, M. (2004) The psychosocial aspects of children exposed to war: practice and policy initiatives. *Journal of Clinical Psychiatry* 45: 41–62.

Beck, A.T. and Freeman, A. (1990) *Cognitive Therapy of Personality Disorder.* New York: Guildford Press.

Bera, W.H. (1993) Betrayal: clergy sexual abuse and male survivors. *Dulwich Centre Newsletter,* 3–4. In J. Gonsiorek, *Breach of Trust: Sexual Exploitation by Health Care Professionals and Clergy.* London: Sage, 1995.

Bisson, J. and Andrew, M. (2007) Psychological treatment of post traumatic stress disorder (PTSD). *Cochrane Database of Systematic Reviews,* 3.

Blum, W. (2007) *Killing Hope: US Military and CIA Interventions since World War II.* Monroe, ME: Common Courage Press.

Bracken, P.J. (2002) *Trauma: Culture, Meaning and Philosophy.* London: Whurr.

Brandsford, J.D. and Johnson, M.K. (1972) Contextual prerequisites for understanding: some investigations of comprehension and recall. *Journal of Verbal Learning and Verbal Behaviour* 11: 717–26.

Brewin, C.R. and Holmes, E.A. (2003) Psychological theories of posttraumatic stress disorder. *Clinical Psychology Review,* 23: 339–76.

Briere, J. (1996) *Therapy for Adults Molested: Beyond Survival.* New York: Springer.

Bruner, J.S. and Postmand, L. (1949) Perception, cognition, and behaviour. *Journal of Personality,* 18: 206–23.

Centre for Disease Control and Prevention (2003) Costs of Intimate Partner Violence against Women in the United States, April 2003. http://www.nrcdv.org/docs/Mailings/2004/NRCDVDec2004.pdf [accessed 9/09/07].

de Vries, H. (1996) *Philosophy and the Turn to Religion.* Baltimore: Johns Hopkins University Press.

Donaldson, N.A. and Gardner, R. (1985) Diagnosis and treatment of traumatic stress around women after childhood incest. In C.R. Figley (1985) *Trauma and its Wake: The Study and Treatment of Post Traumatic Stress Disorder.* New York: Bruner/Mazel.

Dyrerov, A. and Raundlen, M. (2005) Norwegian adolescents' reactions to distant warfare. *Behavioural Cognitive Psychotherapy,* 33: 443–57.

Ehlers, A. and Clarke, D.M. (2000) A cognitive model of PTSD. *Behaviour Research and Therapy,* 38: 319–45.

Ettinger, L. (1980) *Concentration Camp Syndrome and its Late Sequelae in Survivors, Victims and Perpetrators.* New York: Hemispheres, pp. 127–62.

Farrell, D. P. (2003) Idiosyncratic Trauma Characteristics Experienced by Survivors of Sexual Abuse Perpetrated by Clergy or Religious. PhD thesis, Manchester Metropolitan University.

Flaccus, G. (2007) Los Angeles judge approves $660 million clergy abuse settlement. *Associated Press USA.* FCN Publishing.

Foa, E.B., Keane, T.M., and Friedman, M.J. (2000) Guidelines for the treatment of PTSD. *Journal of Traumatic Stress,* 13: 4, 539–55.

Fortune, M. (1995) Is nothing sacred? In J. Gonsiorek (1995) *Breach of Trust: Sexual Exploitation by Health Care Professionals and Clergy.* London: Sage.

Green, B.L. and Solomon, S.D. (1995) The mental health impact of natural and technological disasters. In J.R. Freedy and S.E. Hobfoll (eds) *Traumatic Stress: From Theory to Practice.* New York: Plenum Press.

Heise, L., Ellsberg, M., and Gottemoeller, M. (1999) *Ending Violence against Women. Population Reports, Series No 11*, December. Baltimore, MD: Johns Hopkins University School of Public Health.

Herman, J.L. (2001) *Trauma and Recovery*. New York: Harper Collins.

Hodgkinson, P.E. and Stewart, M. (1991) *Coping with Catastrophe*. London: Routledge.

Hollon, S.D. and Garber, J. (1988). Cognitive therapy. In: L.Y. Abramson (ed.) *Social Cognition and Clinical Psychology*. New York: Guilford Press, pp. 204–53.

Horowitz, M.J. (1975) Intrusive and repetitive thoughts after stress. *Archives of General Psychiatry*, **32**: 1457–63.

Horowitz, M.J. (1976) *Stress Response Syndromes*. New York: Jason Aronson.

Horowitz, M.J. (1986a) *Stress Response Syndromes*. New Jersey: Jason Aronson.

Horowitz, M.J. (1986b) Stress response syndromes: a review of post -traumatic and adjustment disorders. *Hospital and Community Psychiatry*, **37**: 241–9.

International Strategy for Disaster Reduction (2004) World Disaster Reduction Campaign. http://www.unisdr.org/eng/public_aware/world_camp/2004/pa-camp04-inter-day-eng. htm [accessed 10/09/07].

Janet, P. (1989) L'automatisme psychologique (1899) and Nevroses et idées fixes (1898). In C. Caruth (ed.) *Trauma: Explorations in Memory*. Baltimore, MD: Johns Hopkins University Press.

Janoff-Bulman, R. (1985) The aftermath of victimisation: rebuilding shattered assumptions. In C.R. Figley (ed.) *Trauma and its Wake: Vol. 1*. New York: Brunner/Mazel, pp. 15–35.

Janoff-Bulman, R. (1992) *Shattered Assumptions: Towards a New Psychology of Trauma*. New York: The Free Press.

Jehu, D., Klassen, C., and Gazan, M. (1986) Cognitive restructuring of distorted beliefs associated with childhood sexual abuse. *Journal of Social Work and Human Sexuality*, **4**: 25–45.

Kardiner, A. and Speigel, H. (1947) *War Stress and Neurotic Illness* (later revised as *The Traumatic Neurosis of War*). New York: Hober.

Kennerley, H. (1996) Cognitive therapy of dissociative symptoms associated with trauma. *British Journal of Clinical Psychology*, **53**: 325–40.

Kilpatrick, D.G., Veronen, L.J., and Resick, P.A. (1982) Psychological sequelae to rape: assessment and treatment strategies. In D.M. Doleys (ed.) *Behaviour Medicine: Assessment and Treatment Strategies*. New York: Plenum.

King, M.L. (1965) A letter from Birmingham Jail 16 April 1963. In *Why We can't Wait*. New York: Penguin (reissued 2000).

Langer, L.L. (1991) *Holocaust Testimonies: The Ruins of Memory*. New Haven: Yale University Press.

Loughrey, G.C., Bell, P., Kee, M., Roddy, R.J., and Curran, P.S. (1988) PTSD and civil violence in Northern Ireland. *British Journal of Psychiatry*, **153**: 554–60.

Mayou, R., Bryant, B., and Duthie, R. (1993) Psychiatric consequences of road traffic accidents. *British Medical Journal*, **307**: 647–51.

McCann, I.L. and Pearlman, L.A. (1990) *Psychological Trauma and the Adult Survivor: Theory, Therapy, and Transformation*. New York: Bruner/Mazel.

McCann, I.L., Sakheim, D.K., and Abrahamson, D.J. (1988) Trauma and victimisation: a model of psychological adaptation. *The Counselling Psychologist*, **16**: 531–94.

Montazeri, A. and Baradaran, H. (2005) Psychological distress among Bam earthquake survivors in Iran: a population based study. *BMC Public Health*, **5**(1): 4.

NICE (National Institute for Clinical Excellence) (2005) *The Management of Post-Traumatic Stress Disorder (PTSD) in Adults and Children in Primary and Secondary Care*. London: HMSO.

O'Brien, M. and Nutt, D. (1998) Loss of consciousness and post-traumatic stress disorder: a clue to aetiology and treatment. *British Journal of Psychiatry*, **173**: 102–4.

OECD European Conference of Ministers of Transport (2006) *Working Group on Achieving Ambitious Road Safety Targets*. Joint Organisation for Economic Co-operation and Development/ECMT Transport Research Centre.

Piaget, J. (1973) *Structuralism*. New York: Basic Books.

Resick, P.A. and Schnicke, M.K. (1990) Treating symptoms in adult victims of sexual assault. *Journal of Interpersonal Violence*, 5: 488–506.

Resick, P.A. and Schnicke, M.K. (1993) *Cognitive Processing for Rape Victims*. Thousand Oaks, CA: Sage.

Shapiro, F. (1989) Eye movement desensitisation: A new treatment for PTSD. *Journal of Behaviour Therapy and Experimental Psychiatry*, 20: 211–17.

Shapiro, F. (1995) *Eye Movement Desensitisation and Reprocessing, Basic Principles, Protocols and Procedures*. New York: Guildford Press.

Shapiro, F. (2001) *Eye Movement Desensitisation and Reprocessing, Basic Principles, Protocols and Procedures* (2nd edn). New York: Guildford Press.

Sherry, D.F. and Shacter, D.L (1987) The evolution of multiple memory systems. *Psychological Review*, 94(4): 439–54.

Smucker, M.R. (2004) Assessing, predicting, and overcoming treatment road blocks with complex PTSD: developing CBT interventions in accordance with specific trauma characteristics. Paper presented at the EABCT Conference, Manchester.

Smucker, M.R., Dancu, C., Foa, E.B., and Niederee, J.L. (1995) Imagery rescripting: a new treatment for survivors of child sexual abuse suffering from PTSD. *Journal of Cognitive Psychotherapy: An International Quarterly*, 9(1): 3–17.

Spiers, T. and Harrington, G. (2001) *Trauma: A Practitioner's Guide to Counselling*. Hove: Brunner-Routledge.

van der Kolk, B.A. (1996) The body keeps the score: approaches to psychobiology of PTSD. In B.A. van der Kolk, A.C. McFarlane, and L. Weisaeth (eds) *Traumatic Stress: The Effects of Overwhelming Experience on Mind, Body and Society*. New York: Guildford Press.

van der Kolk, B.A., Boyd, G.H., and Krystal, J. (1985) Inescapable shock, neurotransmitters and addition to trauma: towards a psychobiology of PTSD. *Biological Psychiatry*, 20: 314–25.

van der Kolk, B.A., Spinazzola, J., Blaustein, M.E., Hopper, J.W., Hopper, E.K., Korn, D.L., and Simpson, W.B. (2007) A randomised clinical trial of eye movement desensitisation and reprocessing (EMDR), flouxetine and pill placebo in the treatment of post-traumatic stress disorder: treatment effects and long-term maintenance. *Journal of Clinical Psychiatry*, 68: 1 January.

van der Kolk, B.A. and van der Hart, O. (1995) The intrusive past: the flexibility of memory and the engraving of trauma. In C. Caruth (ed.) *Trauma: Explorations in Memory*. Baltimore, MD: Johns Hopkins University Press.

WHO (World Health Organization) (2007) Road traffic crashes leading cause of death in young Europeans. http://www.euro.who.int/mediacentre/PR/2007/20070420_1 [accessed 08/09/07].

Williams, R. (2006) The psychosocial consequences for children and young people who are exposed to terrorism, war, conflict and natural disasters. *Current Opinions Psychiatry*, 19(4): 337–47.

Williams, R.M. and Yule, W. (1988) *The Assessment of 'Nervous Shock' in Compensation Litigation*. London: Sage.

Wilson, J.P. and Keane, T. (2004) *Assessing Psychological Trauma and PTSD*. London: Guildford Press.

World News (2007) US military deaths in Iraq surpass 9/11 toll. www.msnbc.msn.com/id/16356321/ [accessed 29/01/08].

Young, A. (1995) *The Harmony of Illusions: Inventing PTSD*. Princeton, NJ: Princeton University Press.

Young, J.E. (1990) *Cognitive Therapy for Personality Disorders: A Schema-Focused Approach*. Sarasota, FL: Professional Resource Exchange.

Young, J.Z. (1987) *Philosophy and the Brain*. Oxford: Oxford University Press.

Yule, W. (2000) *Post-Traumatic Stress Disorders: Concepts and Therapy*. Chichester: Wiley.

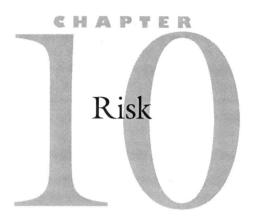

Risk

Tim Turner and Anthony Colombo

BRIEF CHAPTER OUTLINE

This chapter aims to provide a critical exploration of risk within the context of mental health practice. Commencing with risk and insecurity, a sociological context is used as a means of identifying the rapid social changes of the twentieth century and the origins of the risk agenda. This section is followed by politics of exclusion via the label of dangerous severe personality disorder (DSPD). The science of risk assessment then highlights the use of actuarial risk calculations influencing health, social and criminal justice agencies. Next, the illusion of applying the tenets of natural science to the interpretation of human action is discussed; also, efficacy and function of the risk tools used. The chapter ends by examining positive risk-taking.

Introduction

There is little doubt that the twin concepts of risk assessment and risk management now dominate the foreground of the contemporary mental health landscape. Professionals from key agencies routinely utilize an array of tools to measure the risk of all those who pass through their field of vision. Indeed the notion of *risk*, as the central hub from which all else flows, has arguably displaced *care* as the defining purpose of service-user contact. This situation is so deeply embedded within the mental health system that it is rarely reflected upon in any meaningful way. This chapter aims to provide a critical exploration of risk within mental health practice. The outline of the chapter invites mental health practitioners to reflect on their role as risk assessors, particularly in terms of *context* (what are the origins of the risk agenda?), *efficacy* (how accurate are risk judgements?), *function* (what purpose does risk assessment fulfil?) and *impact* (what affect does the risk agenda have on the relationship between practitioners and service users?)

Risk and insecurity: the sociological context

The key to understanding the centrality of risk in current mental health practice lies in the rapid transformation of western society over the last fifty years or so. The post-war period of the late 1940s was a world characterized by fixed social narratives and absolutist standards. Mobility was fairly limited for the majority of society; people invariably spent their lives in the communities they were born within, constrained by the confines of the class system. Common community values prevailed and were rarely questioned. Teenagers of the time were little more than miniature versions of their parents, destined to tread similar pathways through life. Prosperity was on the ascendancy and society seemed to concur to a moral, 'taken-for-granted' consensus. As capitalism, consumerism and industrialization gathered pace, the great western liberal democracies were considered to be arriving at the logical pinnacle of human development (Young, 1999).

This world of modernity was, however, soon to become fractured. A cultural revolution began to ferment during the 1950s and then exploded during the 1960s. Values that had appeared fixed and absolute were suddenly contorted within a kaleidoscope of pluralism. In the new late modern landscape social dimensions that had once provided a solid narrative template (i.e. gender, class, race) were transformed as individuals became free to construct their own interpretations of sub-cultural identity (Hobsbawm, 1994; Young, 1999, 2004). Seats of power, traditionally uncontested, were assaulted across numerous fronts by an array of protest movements. The shackles of gender were unlocked by the rise of feminism. The endemic racism that permeated society was countered by swelling civil rights campaigns and US citizens poured on to the streets to protest against the Vietnam War.

The rapid social changes that occurred during this time and over the latter third of the twentieth century resulted in what Young (2004: 14) has termed a 'loosening of the moorings'. The ontological security that flowed from modernist absolutism became ruptured by massive cultural transformation. Pluralistic values emanating from immigration and subculture essentially made absolute standards impossible to maintain. Globalization and a mass population movement meant a blurring of cultural boundaries as the demarcation between nations became less distinct. The bedrock of modernity, the family, was transformed into a myriad of structural variations and material security was undermined, as 'jobs for life' became obsolete.

The pluralistic, late modern world is therefore full of uncertainty. Individuals throughout the class structure experience a destabilizing ontological insecurity that flows from broken narratives. The fragmented inner cities of the twenty-first century are unrecognizable from the solid communities of post-war modernity. As society has become increasingly atomized, fellow-citizens are viewed with suspicion and strangers become sources of fear. In the urban sprawl, neighbours function in isolation despite their stifling proximity (Godin, 2006: Young, 1999).

While anxiety permeates relationships at the micro-level of society, uncertainty and insecurity also occur at the macro-level as the populations of advanced industrial societies grapple with what Beck (1992) terms a risk consciousness. Such risk preoccupation is focused upon the plethora of new dangers created by the process of industrialization. Thus the nineteenth-century scientific developments that sought to make risk calculable paradoxically led to the inception of a whole range of new hazards. Consequently while the disasters of the pre-modern era were invariably construed as divine acts (acts of God) that could not have been prevented, such catastrophes are now viewed as the inextricable by-products of industrialization. In this context, events like the Chernobyl disaster and the South-East Asian tsunami are seen as firm evidence of the folly of industrial and technological advancement. While risk has always been an inexorable aspect of life, the risk of late modernity differs in the respect that it is humans who are cast as the principal agents of its creation. Such a process has resulted in a widespread distrust of experts as the assurances of science have become undermined and brought into question (Beck, 1992: Fulcher and Scott, 2003: Giddens, 1991: Godin, 2006). The late modern world is therefore characterized by insecurity and uncertainty at both the micro- and macro-level. It is, to quote Giddens (1999), a 'runaway world' that engenders little sense of control over one's own destiny.

Such endemic societal insecurity resulted in a significant transformation of both public and political attitudes towards crime, law and order over the latter stages of the twentieth century. As the crime rate continued to rise across western democracies, public anxiety escalated to new levels as risk avoidance and crime control became increasingly politicized (Beck, 1992; Stenson and Edwards, 2001). In this context the concepts of punishment and control began to converge and the boundary between coercive and non-coercive social control became increasingly difficult to decipher (Garland, 2001: Hudson, 2003). In this 'exclusive' society (Young, 1999) the locus of crime control, previously dominated by the police, became dispersed among numerous key agencies of control, particularly probation, psychiatry and social work (Rose, 2000). The new vision was of a social control that extended far beyond the walls of the prison, an expanding panoptic net of coercion that would enable the state to know all. In the seminal *Visions of Social Control,* Cohen (1985: 85) identifies the role of social workers and psychiatrists in executing 'suffocating layers of community control, camouflaged by mellifluous "psychobabble".'

The state's emphasis therefore became the incapacitation of offenders through dispersed systems of control which were organized at a distance and which embraced risk as a central component (Garland, 2001). This process has been described as indicative of a new penology that moves away from individual notions of dangerousness to exert control over whole population groups

(Feeley and Simon, 1992, 1994). This is achieved by networks of allied agencies engaging systems of surveillance to monitor individuals who have been subjected to actuarial risk aggregation to predict the likelihood of future offending. The efficacy of actuarialism will be considered further on within this chapter.

The principal remit of key agencies has therefore been transformed under the new penology. The focus has switched from one of reformation and rehabilitation to one of control and incapacitation. Probation, for example, has moved from a welfare-driven service aiming to befriend offenders to one that places public protection at its epicentre (Kemshall, 1998). Thus, the welfare function of such agencies has been distorted by a focus on risk that has little to do with rehabilitation. As Garland (2001: 176) argues:

> Where rehabilitative interventions are undertaken today their character is rather different than before. Their focus is more upon issues of crime control than upon individual welfare, and are more 'offence centred' than 'client-centred'...The immediate point is no longer to improve the offender's self-esteem, develop insight, or deliver client-centred services, but instead to impose restrictions, reduce crime, and protect the public.

The change of focus for these professional groups arguably makes their principal function the exertion of a covert and far-reaching form of crime control underpinned by an omnipresent 'risk gaze' (Rose, 2000: 335). In this sense, a pervasive network of subtle surveillance bolsters the thin blue line of the police service. Although such monitoring is frequently disguised as benevolent in nature, on a macro-level, there is little doubt that the primary aim of psychiatry and allied agencies is the control and exclusion of deviance (Godsi, 1999).

While the risk agenda is therefore a dominant aspect of current mental health practice, critics argue that this has little to do with the best interests of service users. Rather, risk facilitates the control of the difficult individuals society has come to view with decreasing tolerance in late modernity (Young, 1999; 2007). Such punitive public attitudes are particularly evident in the aftermath of high-profile homicides. One tragic incident in particular was to become the catalyst to a politics of exclusion that embraced risk as the means of facilitating both preventative detention and eventually the introduction of Indeterminate Public Protection sentences (IPP) (Home Office, 2003) for the dangerous classes.

Risk and the politics of exclusion

Mental health practitioners face the frequent ethical predicament of balancing the rights of service users against an increasingly stringent public protection agenda. In the current context of the new penology and the burgeoning risk agenda, the balance that has been inexorably edging towards social control finally tipped when Michael Stone murdered Linn Russell and her young daughter Megan, in 1996.

This double homicide occurred against a backdrop of concern about a dangerous group of individuals who sat interstitially between services. The highly complex, ill-defined needs and frequently high-risk behaviour of these individuals meant that most agencies, including psychiatry, tried to distance themselves from any sense of accountability. However, Stone's past contact with various social and psychiatric services pushed the issue of dangerous offenders to the top of the political agenda. As the culture of welfare yielded to the culture of control, the public's fear of indiscriminate violence seemed to have reached saturation point (Farnham and James, 2001; Maguire and Bookman, 2005).

Such public demands for more punitive public protection measures were frequently aired through the conduit of the mass media. The murder of Sarah Payne by sex offender Roy Whiting in 2000, for example, led to a high-profile newspaper campaign for the introduction of a Sarah's Law (based upon Megan's Law in the United States) which would give the public access to the Sex Offenders' Register for the first time (Hudson, 2003).

This punitive turn led to the birth of the highly contested, political construction of 'dangerous and severe personality disorder' (Home Office and DH, 1999). In brief, these proposals indicated the introduction of preventative detention and indeterminate sentences for individuals deemed to represent a high risk of violence to the public. Such decisions would utilize actuarial risk assessment to create an 'archipelago of confinement without reformation' (Rose, 2000: 335). The fact that politicians, rather than psychiatrists, had constructed the DSPD label in a populist attempt to facilitate the incapacitation of the allegedly dangerous seemed of little concern to the majority of the public.

Whether or not such individuals should be detained under the umbrella of mental health services is widely contested. However, it is of little surprise that violence, like so many other aspects of life, should become medicalized. This in itself does not represent a shift in ideology but further evidence of the seeping encroachment of the therapeutic state (Cohen, 1985, Godsi, 1999). The political construction of DSPD as a *medical* problem rather than a *social* problem therefore conveniently closes the legal loophole that permits the law to intervene only *after* a crime has been committed (Mullen, 2007). In order to achieve this, those previously deemed untreatable are magically transformed as treatable, despite the stark lack of any new evidence.

The DSPD project and wider proposals have been met with scepticism from user groups and practitioners alike (Tyrer, 2002). Critique focuses predominantly on the complex ethical issues that are associated with such proposals. Detaining individuals for offences that they have yet to commit contradicts the very essence of the western legal system and raises major moral questions regarding human rights. The question as to when individuals would no longer be considered 'dangerous' appears to be vague. Indeed the unlawful nature of the recently introduced IPP has been exposed, as prisoners have been released in the absence of the rehabilitative measures required to reduce their risk (Guardian Online, 2007b).

Critics of the DSPD construct also articulate concerns regarding the stigma of such a powerful label. While the project holds up community reintegration as a long-term aim, the likelihood of ever shedding the DSPD label is surely remote. Such a label should, however, be viewed within the context of a penal repertoire that actively embraces the stigmatization of offenders (Garland, 2001:181). Where shame and stigma were once deemed harmful to the prisoner's self-esteem, the criminal justice system of late modernity exploits shame as a renewed form of punishment. As a result, sex offenders are placed on a register, adolescents are labelled with Anti Social Behaviour Orders (ASBOs), train-fare dodgers are named on posters and shoplifters are paraded in glass cages in a contemporary version of the stocks (Guardian Online, 2007a).

While critics are therefore right to highlight the damaging impact of the DSPD label, they miss the point. This is a deliberate exclusionary stigmatization that serves to alert the wider community to the dangerousness of the individual, just as sex offenders in America must display their predatory presence to a vindictive public. As Jock Young succinctly points out, 'in the late modern world we are not interested in understanding trouble; we simply want to avoid it' (Young, 2007).

Actuarialism: the science of risk assessment

This process of exclusion does, of course, place risk construction firmly at the centre of decision making. In the past, mental health practitioners and allied professionals relied almost entirely on intuition, experience and individual judgement to make these risk-based decisions. The process was more artistic than scientific. While such decisions were often founded on long therapeutic relationships with the people concerned, such intuitive decision-making has since been shown to be highly subjective, unreliable and largely inaccurate (Doyle and Dolan, 2002; Hart, Michie and Cooke, 2007). In the drive for evidence-based practice, a more objective and reliable form of risk assessment was sought. This emerged with the development of actuarial risk assessment instruments (ARAIs), an approach utilized successfully by the insurance industry for many years and which now forms a principal conduit to social control in late modernity (Feeley and Simon, 1992, 1994; Hart and Kirby, 2004; Kemshall, 2003). Such instruments were constructed by statistically analysing the correlates of violent behaviour across wide population groups. Individuals presenting with particular attributes and characteristics could then be mapped on to a risk continuum to gauge the likelihood of them committing future violent acts. Actuarial approaches therefore concern themselves with notions of probability and harm reduction rather than any analysis of causal factors (Young, 1999). It is a process that deliberately disengages practitioners in order to eliminate the problems of inter-rater reliability that had been associated with unstructured clinical judgement.

Actuarial risk calculations therefore became increasingly important to the decisions made by a range of health, social and criminal justice agencies. Such a process corresponded with the ethos of the new penology that saw a departure away from individual constructions of dangerousness. Instead, a more utilitarian mode of justice emerged where the aggregated *probability* of future risk triggers the exclusion of a group of individuals deemed *potentially* too dangerous to participate in free society. This is achieved by assigning the individual to a socially constructed sub-category of risk (e.g. low, medium, high) based upon the convergence of both fixed and dynamic variables (Feeley and Simon, 1992, 1994; Matthews, 2003). Individuals then slide up and down the risk continuum as their circumstances change: although emphasis on static variables, such as previous offending history, makes any significant movement difficult to achieve (Quinsey *et al.*, 1998). Risk assessment in this sense is transformed into a detached, dynamic and pseudo-scientific process. A powerful and objective system that both justifies and facilitates the exclusion and segregation of 'outsiders' deemed, on the basis of perceived attributes, too dangerous to participate in 'normal' society (Garland, 2001; Pratt, 2002).

Risk and the illusion of science

The new penology has been characterized by the introduction of measures such as IPP and preventative detention. Such measures are indicative of a system designed to incapacitate both offenders and potential offenders and which utilizes the statistical analysis of ARAIs as scientific justification to exclude difficult groups of individuals (Hart *et al.*, 2007; Young, 1999). The arbitrary nature of exclusion is therefore eliminated, as the process is transformed into an apparently objective, reliable and scientific process. The decision becomes based upon a value-free statistical equation rather than subjective judgement.

The move towards a more scientific, evidence-based approach to risk is an essential component of the new penology. Thus the key agencies of social control exert the belief that natural scientific methods can be utilized to objectively predict and describe human behaviour. In this sense human action is construed as predetermined and quantifiable (Young, 2004). The scientific validity of actuarial risk assessment is, however, open to critique.

First, applying the tenets of natural science to the interpretation of human action is highly contentious. Humans, unlike natural elements, are not compelled to act in predetermined ways (Hart and Kirby, 2004). Decisions emanate from a complex range of variables and may appear to have no objective sense of rationality. In this context, the algebra of actuarialism is blind to the phenomenology of violence with all its underlying adrenaline, pleasure, excitement, desperation and rage (Young, 2004).

On this basis, the science underpinning actuarial risk assessment becomes illusionary. Furthermore, the veneer of neutrality only disguises a decision-making process that is often founded on subjective judgements about race, gender, class, age and past history (Hannah-Moffat, 1999; Matthews, 2003). The mask of science therefore transforms the high-stake and arguably unethical move towards IPP and preventative detention into a sterile, value-free process.

Secondly, the scientific reliability of actuarial risk assessment is debatable. Put simply, do such instruments yield the same result when different professionals complete them? Anyone with experience of the turbulent dynamics of multi-disciplinary teams will confirm that concurrence is often difficult to establish. Disagreements regarding risk frequently occur between professionals as a result of misaligned values of competing agencies (Timmermans and Gabe, 2001; Turner and Colombo, 2007). The sheer range of ARAIs in circulation only serves to compound this misalignment. The key agencies and professional groups tend to employ their own idiosyncratic choice of ARAI and, as such, draw upon different constellations of variables to assess risk (Doyle and Dolan, 2002; Matthews, 2003). Whilst multi-agency working would undoubtedly be enhanced by a more standardized approach to risk assessment, this would be difficult to establish as the key agencies of social control conceptualize and interpret risk in very different ways. Therefore, although effective multi-agency communication is a cornerstone of the public protection agenda, the conflicting value systems of the professionals concerned means they essentially converse with one another in different languages (Turner and Colombo, 2007). Such different approaches and interpretations of risk undoubtedly have a destabilizing effect on the reliability of risk measurement.

Thirdly, the use of actuarial tools to predict risk at an individual level is highly problematic (Langan and Lindlow, 2004). The design of ARAIs is founded upon statistical probability associated with certain population *groups*; they are indicative only of population trends. Their application to *individuals* is therefore seriously flawed in terms of the margins of error involved. Indeed their use in any form of high-stake decision-making (such as indeterminate sentencing, for example) is essentially unethical (Mullen, 2007). This view is supported by Hart, Michie and Cooke (2007), who evaluated the precision of two commonly used ARAIs: the Violence Risk Appraisal Guide (VRAG) and the Static-99. Results revealed both instruments to be very poor predictive instruments. Indeed, when such instruments are utilized to assess the risk of individuals the results become virtually meaningless. In this sense, the frequent reliance on such instruments by expert witnesses in court is highly contentious and makes such evidence potentially inadmissible. 'As soon as questions of will or decision or reason or choice of action arise, human science is at a loss' (Naom Chomsky, 1978, cited in Swainson, 2000).

The removal of the scientific veneer that coats actuarial risk assessment obviously has significant implications for mental health practice. First and foremost, practitioners must reflect on the function of actuarial risk tools. Are they principally a function of care or control? In the litigious world of mental health practice, such tools give practitioners a sense of expertise and offer some comfort in the knowledge that they have 'done the risk assessment'. However, if the results of such instruments are as meaningless as Hart *et al.* (2007) claim, what are the ethical implications of incorporating them within what should be individualized mental health care packages?

The scientific certainty that is often afforded to actuarial approaches to risk also has obvious implications for the human rights of mental health-service users. In such a utilitarian model, many individuals are likely to lose their liberty under erroneous visions of future violence. Sterile scientific terminology portrays such individuals as *false positives*, a term that does little to capture the sense of injustice that such individuals must experience. Indeed, Buchanan and Leese (2001) suggest that six people with DSPD would have to be detained in order to prevent one violent act. The accuracy of risk assessment is obviously essential if the incidence of false positives is to be kept to a minimum. However, the predictive accuracy of risk judgements is a highly contentious issue.

The drive for evidence-based practice demands that contemporary mental health professionals make informed decisions about risk. The subjectivity of clinical judgement means that actuarial risk assessment tools are frequently used to bolster the decision-making process. Although such instruments have already been described as flawed at the individual level, there is also a danger that such instruments engender a false sense of expertise within practitioners, particularly those who are perhaps less experienced.

Actuarialism essentially reduces individuals to a range of inconsistent variables encompassed within a series of tick boxes. For the practitioner conducting the assessment, a degree of expertise is engendered with the completion of the ARAI. The pseudo-scientific nature of this process is undoubtedly seductive. The sphere of contemporary mental health practice means that accountability and fear of failure weigh heavily in the decision-making process, as the spectre of blame and litigation looms in the background (Godin, 2006). A completed actuarial risk assessment can therefore offer practitioners what is often a false sense of security. ARAIs themselves do not create experts. Effective risk assessment is entirely dependent on the completeness of records, the skill and thoroughness of the interviewer and perhaps, most importantly, the degree to which the interviewee is prepared to disclose information (Quinsey *et al.*, 1998).

While ARAIs therefore go some way in satiating the evidence-based practice agenda they do little to capture the complexity of human action. Individuals interpret the world around them through idiosyncratic lenses; it is this interpretation that governs action and reaction. Thus the delusions of psychosis are embedded within layers of social meaning as individuals strive to make sense of their experiences. When practitioners make predictions about future risk based upon the variables of actuarialism they neglect the phenomenological cultural meanings that govern human action (Ferrell and Sanders, 1995; Young, 2004). The ability of practitioners to identify the relatively small group of individuals who will go on to commit a serious violent offence at some unspecified point in the future is therefore limited. The fact that every risk assessment tool currently in existence yields an inordinately high level of false positives is an indication of the enormity of this task. Human action cannot be reduced to a series of tick boxes. It is infinitely more complex than the statistical clusters of ARAIs.

Towards positive therapeutic risk-taking

So far this chapter has focused on critical aspects of risk within mental health practice. The issue, however, is not one-dimensional. The intention is not to detract from the positive factors that have resulted from a mental health service that has undoubtedly become more proactive and accountable as a result of the risk agenda. This accountability is of course predominantly a result of the inception of the Care Programme approach (CPA) in 1991 (DH, 1990, 2000). The CPA requirement to appoint a key-worker responsible for care co-ordination led to a far more robust and formalized service. The framework also required practitioners to trace the dynamics of risk as regular multi-agency review became embedded within clinical practice.

The need for more stringent approaches to risk and clearer lines of multi-agency communication were of course laid bare with the denouement of uncoordinated practice: the killing of Jonathan Zito by Christopher Clunis at a London Underground station in December 1992. It has been well documented that the sporadic care that Clunis experienced was a significant antecedent to the death of Mr Zito (see Ritchie, Dick and Lingham, 1994). Under the guidelines outlined within CPA, risk was to become a more transparent and formal concept distributed across multi-disciplinary teams. As a result of more robust risk protocols, there have been marked reductions in the number of suicides associated with mental distress and a much greater appreciation of the relationship between mental ill health and vulnerability.

In this sense, it is not the risk agenda in itself that is problematic for service users. Rather it is a narrative that persistently conflates mental ill-health with serious violence (Doyle and Dolan, 2002), despite evidence to the contrary (Taylor and Gunn, 1999). Such views are of course perpetuated by the mass media with clichéd cinematic portrayals of deranged psychopaths and tabloid moral panic over the rare instances of mental illness-related homicide (Clarke, 2004; Cutcliffe and Hannigan, 2001; Hallam, 2002; Stickley and Felton, 2006). Such media coverage does of course seek to scapegoat the experts who failed to act on the warning signs that seem so obvious with all the benefit of hindsight. It is this culture of blame that leads many mental health practitioners into spirals of defensive practice as they anxiously engage in a process of damage limitation.

The increasingly defensive nature of mental health practice is therefore a result of the utopian public perception that *all* risk can and should be eliminated. In this context, an accountability that sits heavily on the shoulders of practitioners ensures that decisions are made on a *worse-case scenario* basis. When the minutiae of client contact are constructed as potential evidence in some imagined future homicide inquiry, the therapeutic nature of engagement is practically nullified. The anxiety that permeates mental health practice therefore creates a context of control and coercion that has little to do with the best interests of service users and which places far too much emphasis on medication compliance (Coleman, 1998). Put simply, this is not a system that supports the positive therapeutic risk-taking that is essential to service users sense of growth and recovery (Langan and Lindow, 2004; Stickley and Felton, 2006).

How then, can practitioners begin to reconstruct risk as a positive catalyst to change and progress? First, it would seem essential to move towards a conception of risk that is founded on partnership with service users. This emphasis on partnership is seen as an 'essential ingredient' of contemporary mental health services (Minett *et al.*, 2005: 9) but is frequently overlooked in the context of risk. In a mental health system that has placed more and more emphasis on the importance of user-focused care, it seems unforgivable that so many service users remain excluded from the management of their own risk. It is essential that service users construe mental health care as a collaborative process (Tummey and Smojkis, 2005); the frequent omission of service users from discussions about their risk status is therefore both unhelpful and unethical. Indeed, even when service users are involved in the process, there is a high level of disagreement in regard to the most appropriate level of risk (Langan and Lindow, 2004).

Clearly this is an important area to address. If risk is to remain at the epicentre of care, it is clearly essential that service users are placed at the core of risk construction. André Gide (1925: cited in Swainson, 2000) stated, 'one doesn't discover new lands without consenting to lose sight of the shore for a very long time.' This will be a requirement if clients themselves are placed at the centre of a needs-based process, allowing practitioners more able to adopt a positive risk-taking strategy that will reap progress and ultimately recovery for the service user. In this sense, individual practitioners need to make defensible rather than defensive decisions in an organizational context that emphasizes positive risk-taking and recovery through clear policies.

If risk is constructed and managed in partnership with service users there is also a strong likelihood that the unrelenting focus on violence will dissipate, as the real risk issues that concern service users come to the fore. Rather than concentrate on the relatively unlikely occurrence of serious violence to others, mental health services may then start to address stigma, poverty, disempowerment and vulnerability, all of which have a significant impact on the lives of those experiencing severe mental ill-health (Pilgrim and Rogers, 1999). The preoccupation with the risk *posed* by those with mental illness is palpably unfair when one considers the high rates of victimization that such individuals endure. While those with mental illness are persistently construed as potential perpetrators of violence, it is ironic that their real contribution to the homicide statistics lies in their high rate of victimization (Hiroeh *et al.*, 2001).

Conclusion

The trusting relationship between mental health practitioners and service users is allegedly at the heart of mental health practice. However, is the need to balance public protection against service users' interests obfuscating the therapeutic nature of this relationship? Mental health practitioners' current role as risk assessors effectively trumps every other aspect of their position. As the lens through which the minutia of every client contact is viewed it creates a frequently insurmountable barrier to therapeutic communication. In this context the practitioner–service user relationship is founded upon a reciprocal context of distrust, suspicion and scepticism.

In a mental health system that allegedly places great emphasis on the importance of engaging reflective practitioners, the role as risk assessors is hardly ever contested or even considered in any meaningful way. Evidence-based practice, likewise, is heralded as a central plank of contemporary practice (Beinecke, 2006), yet the evidence linking mental disorder and violence is, at best, tenuous. Indeed, a recent study by Coid *et al.* (2007) identifies history of violence, gender, age and personality disorder as more robust predictors of future violence than any clinical variable. That they conclude, without any sense of irony, that the most effective means of reducing risk is to increase psychiatric restrictions is perhaps an indication of the scale of the problem.

In the context of contemporary mental health care the risk obsession sits very awkwardly with more progressive political developments. The role of service users, for example, has been increasingly valued in recent years (Campbell, 2005). The acknowledgement of 'expertise through experience' is a welcome departure from past constructions of the service user as a passive recipient of psychiatric expertise. It is now recognized that the experiences of those who have *been there* are a previously untapped source of knowledge. However, as Cohen (1985) points out, some sections of the population can be simultaneously included and excluded by society and consequently the same political party may develop policies that seem to contradict and oppose one another within a relatively short period of time (Pratt, 2002). In this case, then, strategies have been constructed to assert the civil rights of service users and tackle stigma and discrimination (NIMHE, 2004). The impact of such measures has then been negated by populist draconian measures such as the draft Mental Health Bill for England and Wales that serve only to ratchet up public fear and perpetuate stigma and myth.

However, in the late modern context of our risk-averse society, it would be wholly unrealistic to suggest that we can simply dispense with our role as risk assessors. Instead, what is required is a cultural shift in the negative construction of risk, both within the mental health system itself and in the wider political and public discourse. The current climate of litigation, blame and accountability virtually forces the practice of all mental health professionals into ever-decreasing circles of defensibility. In this sense, the remit to engage in a therapeutic relationship with individuals experiencing mental distress becomes diluted by a cynical need to cover one's back (Turner and Colombo, 2007). Is psychiatry's shift towards the science of risk therefore associated, as Shorter (1997) suggests, with a corresponding loss of caring?

The situation is, however, unlikely to change while homicides committed by those experiencing mental ill-health are constructed as the preventable errors of judgement by experts. There needs to be an acknowledgement that tragedy and risk is an inevitable part of the human experience that cannot be eliminated. Human behaviour, frequently irrational and unpredictable, is governed by a myriad of variables that are beyond the scope of actuarial tools. Individuals experiencing mental distress make a very minor contribution to the homicide statistics; it is time this was acknowledged by mental health services. It is the risks faced by service users themselves that should preoccupy mental health professionals.

As human beings we make hundreds of decisions every day, whether it be choosing the nutritional content of our lunch or deciding upon the best route for the commute to work. Whilst we may not be consciously aware of it, elements of risk are intricately woven throughout every one of these choices. In the absence of risk taking our lives would be reduced to a state of catatonic inertia. Risk taking is a positive process that enables us all to progress. Why then should it be different for those experiencing distressing mental health experiences? The journey to recovery for such individuals is long and made infinitely more arduous by a mental health system that constructs risk as a negative concept to be managed and controlled rather than a positive catalyst to therapeutic change.

Issues of difference

* How do constructions of risk differ in relation to gender?

* How does your interpretation of risk change in relation to a service user's age?

* How can we explain the overrepresentation of black people within the secure mental health system?

Relevance to practice

* Do mental health practitioners make defensive or defensible decisions? Reflect on your own practice, with recent examples.

* What are the ethical implications of mental health practitioners sharing risk information with the police?

* What measures can be implemented to make the risk assessment / management process more service user-focused?

Investigate

* What factors influence the accuracy of risk assessment?

* To what extent is it possible to attain a multi-agency standardized approach to risk assessment?

* What are the barriers to effective multi-agency working in regard to risk?

Suggested further reading

Godin, P. (ed.) (2006) *Risk in Nursing Practice*. Basingstoke: Palgrave Macmillan.
Kemshall, H. (2003). *Understanding Risk in Criminal Justice* Berkshire: Open University Press.

References

Beck, U. (1992) *Risk Society: Towards a New Modernity*. London: Sage.
Beinecke, R. (2006) Evidence-based mental health practices. *International Journal of Mental Health* 35(2): 3–5.
Buchanan, A. and Leese, M. (2001) Detention of people with dangerous and severe personality disorders: a systematic review. *The Lancet* **358**: 1955–9.
Campbell, P. (2005) From little acorns: the mental health service user movement. In A. Bell and P. Lindley (eds) *Beyond the Water Towers: The Unfinished Revolution in Mental Health Services 1985–2005*. London: Sainsbury Centre for Mental Health.
Clarke, J. (2004) Mad, bad and dangerous: the media and mental illness. *Mental Health Practice* 7(10): 16–19.
Cohen, S. (1985) *Visions of Social Control*. Cambridge: Polity Press.
Coid, J., Hickey, N., Kahtan, N., Zhang, T. and Yang, M. (2007) Patients discharged from medium secure forensic psychiatry services: reconvictions and risk factors. *British Journal of Psychiatry* **190**: 223–9.

Coleman, R. (1998). *Politics of the Madhouse*. Runcorn: Handsell.

Cutcliffe, J.R. and Hannigan, B. (2001) Mass media, 'monsters' and mental health clients: the need for increased lobbying. *Journal of Psychiatric and Mental Health Nursing* 8(4): 315–21.

DH (1990) *The Care Programme Approach for People with a Mental Illness Referred to the Specialist Psychiatric Services*. HC (90) 23/LASSL (90). London: Department of Health.

DH (2000) *Effective Care Co-ordination in Mental Health Services: Modernising the Care Programme Approach: A Policy Booklet*. London: Department of Health.

Doyle, M. and Dolan, M. (2002) Violence risk assessment: combining actuarial and clinical information to structure clinical judgements for the formulation and management of risk. *Journal of Psychiatric and Mental Health Nursing* 9: 649–57

Farnham, F.R. and James, D.V. (2001) 'Dangerousness' and dangerous law. *The Lancet* **358**: 1926.

Feeley, M. and Simon, J. (1992) The new penology: notes on the emerging strategies of corrections and its implications. *Criminology* 30: 449–74.

Feeley, M. and Simon, J. (1994) Actuarial justice: the emerging new criminal law. In D. Nelken (ed.) *The Futures of Criminology*. London: Sage.

Ferrell, J. and Sanders, C.R. (1995) Culture, crime and criminology. In J. Ferrell and C.R. Sanders, *Cultural Criminology*. Boston: Northeastern University Press

Fulcher, J. and Scott, J. (2003) *Sociology* (2nd edn). Oxford: Oxford University Press.

Garland, D. (2001) *The Culture of Control: Crime and Social Order in Contemporary Society*. Oxford: Open University Press.

Giddens, A. (1991) *Modernity and Self-Identity* Cambridge: Polity Press.

Giddens, A. (1999) Risk and responsibility. *Modern Law Review* **62**(1): 1–10.

Godin, P. (2006) *Risk in Nursing Practice*. Basingstoke: Palgrave Macmillan.

Godsi, E. (1999) *Violence in Society*. London: Constable.

Guardian Online (2007a) Ground floor perfumery, stationery ... and cells. http://www.guardian.co.uk/crime/article/0,2034280,00.html [accessed 15.08.07].

Guardian Online (2007b) Judge warns of danger to public safety after ordering the release of violent offender. http://www.guardian.co.uk/prisons/story/0,2153010,00.html [accessed 12.09.07].

Hallam, A. (2002) Media influences on mental health policy: long term effects of the Clunis and Silcocks cases. *International Review of Psychiatry* **14**(1): 28–33.

Hannah-Moffat, K. (1999) Moral agent or actuarial subject? Risk and Canadian women's imprisonment. *Theoretical Criminology* **3**(1): 71–94.

Hart, D.A. and Kirby, S.D. (2004) Risk prevention. In S.D. Kirby, D.A. Hart, D. Cross and G. Mitchell (eds) *Mental Health Nursing: Competencies for Practice*. Basingstoke: Palgrave Macmillan.

Hart, S.D., Michie, C. and Cooke, D.J. (2007) Precision of actuarial risk assessment instruments: evaluating the 'margins of error' of group v. individual predictions of violence. *British Journal of Psychiatry* **190**(suppl. 49): s60–s65.

Hiroeh, U., Appleby, L., Bo Mortensen, P. and Dunn, G. (2001) Death by homicide, suicide, and other unnatural causes in people with mental illness: a population based study. *The Lancet* **358**: 2110–12.

Hobsbawm, E. (1994) *The Age of Extremes*. London: Michael Joseph.

Home Office (2003) *The Criminal Justice Act*. London: HMSO.

Home Office and DH (1999) *Managing Dangerous People with Severe Personality Disorder*. London: Home Office and Department of Health.

Hudson, B. (2003) *Justice in the Risk Society: Challenging and Re-affirming Justice in Late Modernity*. London: Sage.

Kemshall, H. (1998) *Risk in Probation Practice*. Aldershot: Ashgate.

Kemshall, H. (2003) *Understanding Risk in Criminal Justice*. Maidenhead: Open University Press.

Langan, J. and Lindow, V. (2004) *Living with Risk: Mental Health Service User Involvement in Risk Assessment and Management.* Bristol: Policy Press.

Maguire, M. and Bookman, M. (2005) Violent and sexual crime. In N. Tilley (ed.) *The Handbook of Crime Prevention and Community Safety.* Cullompton: Willan, pp. 516–62.

Matthews, R. (2003) Rethinking penal policy: towards a systems approach. In R. Matthews and J. Young (eds) *The New Politics of Crime and Punishment.* Cullompton: Willan, pp. 223–49.

Minett, R. with Members of the North East Warwickshire User Involvement Project (2005) Partnership with the service user. In R. Tummey (ed.) *Planning Care in Mental Health Nursing.* Basingstoke: Palgrave Macmillan.

Mullen, P.E. (2007) Dangerous and severe personality disorder and in need of treatment. *British Journal of Psychiatry* **190**(suppl. 49): s3–s7.

NICE (2004) *2004–2009: A Strategic Plan to Tackle Stigma and Discrimination on Mental Health Grounds: From Here to Equality.* Leeds: National Institute for Mental Health in England.

Pilgrim, D and Rogers, A. (1999) *A Sociology and Mental Health and Illness* (2nd edn). Buckingham: Open University Press.

Pratt, J. (2002) Critical criminology and the punitive society: some new visions of social control. In K. Carrington and R. Hogg (eds) *Critical Criminology: Issues, Debates, Challenges.* Cullompton: Willan, pp. 185–217.

Quinsey, V.L., Harris, G.F., Rice, M.E. and Cormier, C.A. (1998) *Violent Offenders: Appraising and Managing Risk.* Washington, DC: American Psychological Association.

Ritchie, J.H., Dick, D. and Lingham, R. (1994) *Report of the Inquiry into the Care and Treatment of Christopher Clunis* London: HMSO.

Rose, N. (2000) Government and control. *British Journal of Criminology* **40**(2): 321–9.

Salmi, J. (2004) Violence in democratic societies: towards an analytic framework. In P. Hillyard, C. Pantazis, S. Tombs and D. Gordon (eds) *Beyond Criminology: Taking Harm Seriously.* London: Pluto, pp. 55–66.

Shorter, E. (1997) *A History of Psychiatry: From the Era of the Asylum to the Age of Prozac.* Chichester: Wiley.

Stenson, K. and Edwards, A. (2001) Crime control and liberal government: the 'third way' and the return to the local. In K. Stenson and R.R. Sullivan (eds) *Crime Risk and Justice: The Politics of Crime Control in Liberal Democracies.* Cullompton: Willan, pp. 68–85.

Stickley, T and Felton, A. (2006) Promoting recovery through therapeutic risk taking. *Mental Health Practice* **9**(8): 26–30.

Swainson, B. (ed.) (2000) *Encarta Book of Quotations.* London: Bloomsbury.

Taylor, P. and Gunn, J. (1999) Homicides by people with mental illness: myth and reality. *British Journal of Psychiatry* **174**: 9–14.

Timmermans, S. and Gabe, J. (2001) *Partners in Health, Partners in Crime.* Oxford: Blackwell.

Tummey, R. and Smojkis, M. (2005) Primary mental health care. In R. Tummey (ed.) *Planning Care in Mental Health Nursing.* Basingstoke: Palgrave Macmillan.

Turner, T. and Colombo, A. (2007) Multi-agency public protection panels: can different services ever work together? *Mental Health Practice* **10**(5): 24–5.

Tyrer, P. (2002) Getting to grips with severe personality disorder (Editorial). *Criminal Behaviour and Mental Health* **14**: 1–4.

Young, J. (1999) *The Exclusive Society.* London: Sage.

Young, J. (2004) Voodoo criminology and the numbers game. In J. Ferrell, K. Hayward, W. Morrison and M. Presdee (eds) *Cultural Criminology Unleashed.* London: Glasshouse Press.

Young, J. (2007) *The Vertigo of Late Modernity.* London: Sage.

11

Crime

Anthony Colombo and Tim Turner

BRIEF CHAPTER OUTLINE

The following chapter on crime offers a critical debate on the 'borderland' between mental health and criminal justice. The authors evaluate a range of significant issues that practitioners often take for granted or overlook concerning the offender/patient. A frame of reference is offered through an investigation into who mentally disordered offenders are. Explored through the accessibility of case examples, the chapter unfolds by identifying a number of points and considerations for the reader to ponder. This style is continued through to determine why the medicalization of criminal behaviour is controversial. Another contention is that the sick role may absolve offenders of responsibility. Finally, the chapter raises debate as to whether mentally disordered offenders could ever be viewed as 'normal' and beneficial members of society.

Introduction

Since the latter years of the nineteenth century, two significant assemblages have emerged within western societies in an effort to manage certain forms of behaviour that have come to be considered as socially unacceptable. On the one hand stands the criminal justice system, which is essentially organized around the actions of the police, judiciary, prison and probation services, and whose job it is to deal with deviant individuals defined as 'bad'. On the other stands the mental health system, which employs psychiatrists, psychologists, nurses and therapists in an effort to deal with deviant individuals defined as 'mad'.

Each system may also be differentiated from one another in terms of their underlying rationale. Thus, 'offenders' within the criminal justice process are considered as responsible individuals who are able to exercise free will. Their conduct is judged against parameters set down by the criminal law, the purpose of which is to determine culpability and incarcerate the guilty as a form of punishment for their crimes. Conversely, 'patients' within the mental health service are believed to be 'mentally disordered' and therefore influenced by factors over which they have limited control. Their behaviour is measured against criteria set down specifically for the purpose of making diagnoses, the aim being to provide care in either a hospital or community setting, which administers treatment to the sick.

Such a distinction seems to suggest the existence of two diametrically opposed cultures: the former based on issues concerned with law enforcement and the eradication of crime through punishment; the latter more focused on matters of medicine and the eradication of disease through palliative intervention. In practice, however, these two complex systems occasionally interact and intersect, especially when dealing with 'offenders' who are also considered to be 'mentally disordered'; a population which for many years has been perceived as 'the mad, bad and dangerous to know' (Lamb, 1812).

This point of intersection between the domains of mental health and criminal justice can be likened to a borderland; an area populated by a range of professionals from both systems who come together in order to manage a multitude of situations where legal and medical issues combine (Timmermans and Gabe, 2004). For example, from the standpoint of the 'offender' who is suspected of suffering from mental health difficulties there are at least six critical crossover points within this borderland: (1) at any point after their arrest 'offenders' who are suspected of having a 'mental disorder' can be diverted away from the criminal justice system into the care of mental health and social services (Home Office, 1990); (2) during the pre-trial phase 'offenders' may be found 'unfit to plead', which will result in their detention in a mental hospital without a conviction being recorded (Criminal Procedure (Insanity and Unfitness to Plead) Act, 1991); (3) at the trial offenders can use the legal defence of insanity to claim that their state of mental health was such that they did not know what they were doing at the time of the offence. If successful, a verdict of 'not guilty by reason of insanity' is given and the offender will be detained and treated in hospital rather than punished in prison (McNaughton Rules, 1843); (4) after being convicted of a crime offenders may use evidence of a mental disorder to mitigate the nature of the sentence. For example, a psychiatric probation order may be given instead of custody (Schedule 1:5 Criminal Justice Act, 1991); (5) offenders who become mentally disordered while in prison may be transferred to the mental health system where they can be detained and treated in hospital

(Part III Mental Health Act, 1983); and (6) specialist forensic services now exist for the better management and care of mentally disordered offenders, either within secure provisions or the community (Reed Report, 1992).

The aim of this chapter is to critically evaluate a range of significant issues that practitioners often take for granted or overlook concerning the offender/patient population who occupy the borderland intersecting mental health and criminal justice matters. In particular, our discussion will be organized around three highly divisive questions, namely: Who are mentally disorder offenders? Why is the medicalization of criminal behaviour controversial? And can 'mentally disordered offenders' ever be seen as normal and beneficial members of society?

Who are 'mentally disordered offenders'?

According to the Reed Report (1992), 'mentally disordered offenders' are characterized as people with a 'mental disorder' who have or who are alleged to have broken the criminal law. However, such a definition is unsatisfactory at both the level of social theory and basic science as it tells us nothing about what it actually means to have a 'mental disorder' or to have 'broken the criminal law'. During the course of their daily activities most practitioners probably have little time to give much thought to such concerns, setting aside definitional matters as secondary to getting on with the job in hand. Yet it is important to recognize that the 'problem of defining deviance' is central to resolving the 'deviancy problem' (Mickalowski, 1985). In other words, attempting to make sense of the concepts 'mental disorder' and 'crime' should be viewed as an essential part of practice because the underlying assumptions that we often implicitly make about the nature of the individuals behind these labels is likely to have a fundamental impact on our actions and reactions (Colombo, 1997; Colombo *et al.*, 2003).

Images of deviance: mental disorder, criminal behaviour
and the biomedical model

When someone presents with patterns of abnormality that are non-physical in nature, such as hearing voices or having suicidal ideations, the most dominant response from within psychiatry is to conceptualize these experiences in accordance with the principles of the biomedical approach (Schwartz, 1999; Wakefield, 1992). Thus, it is assumed that such 'disorders of the mind' represent signs and symptoms of some underlying physiological dysfunction or disease located at either the genetic, biochemical or neurological level. For example, several scholars have suggested that schizophrenia may be the result of a neurotransmitter imbalance (McKenna, 1997) or genetic predisposition (Murray, Walsh and Arsenault, 2002), while others have produced research evidence demonstrating that mental disturbances such as Huntington's disease, general paresis and alcoholic poisoning can be clearly understood in terms of an organic pathology (Lishman, 1997).

Furthermore, criminologists have always been interested in the biological basis of criminality (Ellis, 1996; Wilson, 1975). In fact, there exists a growing volume of research which is starting to take seriously the possibility that the origins of various forms of criminal activity such as sexual misconduct, violence and aggression might be rooted in a series of biological anomalies, involving some combination of: genetic, evolutionary, biochemical, toxicological and neurophysiological factors (Williams, 2004). Moreover, the possibility of a link between a person's physiology and their propensity to commit crime has been recognized in legal practice. For example, in England and Wales a woman charged with killing her baby within one year of its birth can appeal to the special defence of *infanticide* if it can be shown that she suffered from postpartum depression syndrome (Infanticide Act, 1938). The case study below also shows that even what you eat may result in biological changes that can influence a person's involvement in criminal conduct:

CASE STUDY I

In 1979 Dan White, a local government official, attacked and killed a work colleague and the Mayor of San Francisco, USA. At his trial, White pleaded not guilty and used as his defence evidence relating to the impact excessive amounts of sugar can have on behaviour. In particular, his lawyers argued that when Mr White got depressed he resorted to eating large volumes of high-sugar junk food such as Twinkies, fizzy drinks and chocolate. Expert testimony at the trial claimed that the large dose of sugar from this junk food used up White's insulin supply which resulted in the body not being able to produce sufficient glucose energy for normal brain functioning. The jury accepted that White's diet had diminished his capacity to control his behaviour and found him guilty of manslaughter rather than murder, for which he was sentenced to prison for 5 years. Mr White's defence has since been referred to as the 'junk-food' or 'Twinkie' defence, though subsequent attempts to use this strategy in court have failed. Shortly after his release Dan White committed suicide.

Thus, at a very basic level it could be argued that human beings are just one of many different organic species living on this planet and the way we behave, how we think and what we feel constitute our existence, which must be rooted in our biological makeup. Moreover, behaviour is still human behaviour no matter what labels we attribute to its various forms: mentally disordered, criminal, deviant, antisocial or normal. On the basis of such an assumption, and the available evidence, it is not such a quantum leap to suggest that there might exist a relationship between specific physiological attributes or anomalies and some forms of mentally abnormal and criminal conduct. In fact, case study 2 clearly indicates a close, albeit complex, association between mental disorder and criminal behaviour when defined within a biomedical framework. As to whether mental disturbance is the cause of crime, or whether crime is evidence (a symptom) of mental disorder remains a moot point:

CASE STUDY 2

Charles Whitman killed his family, and then, from a building overlooking the University of Texas, USA, he used a high-powered rifle to kill 14 people and wound 24 others before being shot by police. An autopsy revealed that Whitman had a malignant brain tumour, which may have been responsible for his violent conduct. The connection was further complicated by evidence from Whitman's own diaries and psychiatric evaluations prior to his crimes, which recorded growing feelings of paranoia and increasing difficulty in trying to control his homicidal urges.

Images of deviance: mental disorder, criminal behaviour
and the biomedical myth

While the biomedical approach generally works well for physical medicine, the analogy does not translate so convincingly for the purposes of defining mental disorders. In fact for most conditions, especially the more prevalent 'functional' disorders, no organic aetiology has been established (Pilgrim and Rogers, 1999). Researchers have also noted that there exists considerable overlap and heterogeneity in the description and classification of apparently medically distinct psychopathological states (Clark, Watson and Reynolds, 1995).

Furthermore, any discussion about 'disorders of the mind' raises complex philosophical questions as to what this actually means (Descartes, 1997). For example, scholars have argued that discussions of the mind, as an entity distinct from the physical brain, are unscientific because the subject matter concerns psychic phenomena too subjective and imprecise for empirical testing (Halfpenny 1982). In other words, there exists no scientific evidence to support the assumption that the mind occupies physical reality; we cannot see it on an X-ray or under a microscope, it has no pulse that we are aware of; it cannot be dissected, or tangibly experienced by our senses in any other way. Consequently, we must conclude that the 'mind' cannot be objectively studied in the same way as physiological conditions; that it is merely an inferential leap of faith, rather than sound scientific judgement, which leads practitioners to presume that abnormal mental experiences are symptomatic of some underlying physical malady. In fact, some scholars have even gone so far as to argue that such a biomedical model analogy is a myth when referring to psychological abnormalities, for how can the mind be diseased when it cannot be shown to positively exist in the first place (Szasz, 1961).

Equally, while there appears to be some interest in biosocial explanations of criminal behaviour, this subject remains at the periphery within mainstream criminology relative to an exploration of social factors (Downes and Rock,

2003). Moreover, recent work on the relationship between neurophysiological abnormalities and violent crime using various forms of computerized scanning technologies such as magnetic resonance imaging (or MRI scan) and brain-imaging methods such as positron emission tomography (PET) have failed to produce convincing results. This conclusion has provoked some scholars to denounce the use of such sophisticated tools as little more than 'digital phrenology', searching for bumps on the inside rather than the outside of the head (Niehoff, 1999). Meanwhile, others who have carried out thorough reviews of the literature describe the contribution of biological factors to crime as 'substantively trivial' (Gottfredson and Hirschi, 1990). In fact, even the microscopic dissection of the brain of a multiple murderer failed to reveal evidence of a biological basis to their criminal behaviour (see case study 3).

CASE STUDY 3

On 10 May 1994 the serial killer John Wayne Gacy, Jr. was executed by lethal injection for the rape and murder of 33 boys and young men. Less than 24 hours after his death, the University of Chicago Medical Centre had obtained approval from Gacy's family and lawyer to carry out a microscopic study of his brain tissue in order to try and find positive evidence of a biological link to crime. In particular, the research team were looking for abnormalities in the anatomical size and structure of certain areas of the brain, signs of viral infection or tumours, birth defects, or other subtler forms of neuropathological damage. Ultimately, the research team had to conclude that they were unable to find any physiological disease of dysfunction that might have helped explain John Gacy's abnormal behaviour.

Images of deviance: mental disorder, criminal behaviour
and the social constructionist model

As there is no positive biomedical basis confirming why certain forms of behaviour should be defined as either mentally disordered or criminal, we must logically conclude that they do not exist as objectively verifiable phenomena. In other words, while physical states of matter such as gases, liquids, rocks and planets can all be scientifically identified and measured directly, there are no patterns of behaviour in existence that are universally accepted as constituting naturally occurring entities which are always referred to as 'mental disorders' or 'crimes'.

Instead, they should be understood as subjective judgements made within the context of elaborate classificatory systems. For mental disorders the two most important texts are the *Diagnostic and Statistical Manual* (*DSM-IV*; APA, 2000), and the *International Classification of Diseases* (*ICD 10*; WHO, 1992), each of which claims to follow a biomedical algorithmic process that helps to determine the classification, aetiology, prognosis and treatment of 'diseases of the mind'. Conversely, crime is usually defined as any form of behaviour in violation of the criminal law (Ormerod, 2005). While the criminal law itself may be understood as 'a body of specific rules regarding human conduct which have been promulgated (written down and distributed) by political authority, which apply uniformly to all members of the classes to which the rules refer (equally to everyone in society), and which are enforced by punishment administered by the state' (Sutherland and Cressey, 1970: 8).

Thus, because human conduct does not possess a series of characteristics that make it naturally identifiable as either a 'mental disorder' or a 'crime', we must rely on labelling patterns of behaviour as such in accordance with the diagnostic or legal rules that each particular society decides to set for itself. In other words, both 'mental disorder' and 'crime' can only exist as socially (rather than scientifically/biomedically) constructed phenomena. This means that what we define as 'mad' or 'bad', our images of deviance, can change dramatically depending on how such labels are applied: to different forms of behaviour, at different times, in different places, and to different people behaving in exactly the same way (Becker, 1963).

Moreover, a range of behaviours once criminalized as detrimental to society have since been made lawful, including holding gold in the house, writing a cheque for less than one dollar, printing books (Sutherland and Cressey, 1970), suicide (Suicide Act, 1961), abortion (Sexual Offences Act, 1967; Sexual Offences Act [Scotland] 2004) and homosexual conduct between consenting adults over the age of 16 (Sexual Offences [Amendment] Act, 2000) Even people whose ideas were at one time condemned by their society as either insane or criminal have subsequently come to be regarded as heroes, including the philosopher Socrates (469–399 BC), who is now considered as one of the wisest men to have ever lived, and Nelson Mandela, who was imprisoned for speaking out against apartheid in South Africa before eventually emerging to become the democratically elected president of his country.

Thus, in the absence of scientific/biomedical certainties regarding the objective nature of human conduct; all that we are left with is subjectivity. Understood in these terms, how people act becomes less important than the way in which different *socially constructed meanings* become attributed to those actions. For example, ending the life of another person against their will would usually be defined as the actions of 'madman' and/or a 'murderer'. However, this outcome is not inevitable: during wartime the military may be labelled as *heroes* for killing the enemy; the State provides itself with the legitimate power to execute some offenders in the name of *punishment*; and we medically and legally justify other forms of taking human life by using various labels such as *accidents, self-defence, infanticide, suicide* and in some countries such as Switzerland, *euthanasia*.

However, a particular challenge to this social constructionist hypothesis has come from various social scientists who have tried to show that some forms of conduct are so 'bad' that they are universally condoned as socially harmful. Moreover, these scholars contend that it is these behaviours that are amenable to scientific study in terms of searching for an underlying psychopathological cause (Sellin, 1938).

Actually, this is an intriguing prospect that we can test for ourselves. Let us start with the most bizarre behaviour that we could possibly imagine, say cannibalism; the killing of another person followed by the consumption of their human flesh. Often this is portrayed in films such as George Romero's *Dawn of the Dead* or Lucio Fulci's *Zombie Flesh Eaters* as something so terrifying and barbaric that surely popular opinion everywhere would always be against such conduct. Yet the case studies presented below clearly illustrate that when we examine popular, medical and legal reactions to such 'mad and bad' behaviour more closely, we often find that the notion of universal disapproval is a great deal more complex than we might ordinarily presume.

CASE STUDY 4

In March 2001 Armin Meiwes, a 42-year-old computer specialist from Rotenburg, confessed to killing, slaughtering and then eating the flesh of Bernd Jürgen Brandes from Berlin. What makes this event even more disturbing is the fact that according to Meiwes the victim had volunteered to his fate by responding to an advertisement placed on a website for enthusiasts of cannibalism (apparently there are dozens of such sites in existence). The legal difficulty arising in this case was that because Brandes had given his consent to be slaughtered, a fact verified by video evidence of the incident, it would be difficult to convict Meiwes of murder, which carries a possible life sentence. Furthermore, because of the rare and unusual nature of the behaviour, Germany, like most other countries, has no laws forbidding cannibalism. Thus, in terms of strict legal theory it could be argued that no significant crime had been committed. Psychiatric evaluations also showed that Armin was not suffering from any mental health problems and that he presented as a rational, insightful person who was always in control of his actions. In the end the defendant was charged with 'disturbing the piece of the dead', which in this case amounted to butchering and devouring (over a period of several months) almost 22 kg of the victim's body, for which he was convicted and sentenced to prison for 8½ years. In his summation Judge Wolker Muetze said that the defendant had not committed murder in the legal sense, 'but a behaviour which is condemned in our society – namely the killing and butchering of a human being'.

But contrast this with the following:

CASE STUDY 5

On 5 July 1884, the crew of a yacht called the Mignonette ran into bad weather 1,600 miles off the Cape of Good Hope, South Africa. The yacht sank, forcing the crew of three men and a cabin boy to put to sea in a small open boat with no supplies of food and little water. After several weeks the men were in a desperate

---

CASE STUDY 5 continued

condition and so agreed to kill the cabin boy as he was very weak. The remaining crew then drank his blood and fed on his body. About four days later they were rescued by a passing ship. It was obvious from the remains of the cabin boy left in the boat what had happened and Dudley, one of the crew who had carried out the killing, freely explained his actions.

When news spread about the rescue everyone was very supportive of the crew and treated them as heroes for having endured such hardship and managing to survive. Even so, Dudley and another crew member, Stevens, were arrested, and tried for murder. At the trial, however, the crew were regarded by the jury as having done nothing wrong, the judge received death threats against him if he dared to convict the men, and during the trial the brother of the dead cabin boy actually stood up for the defence and stated how proud he was that his kin had died in this way and that he did not hold Dudley and the others responsible. Furthermore, it is also alleged that Queen Victoria had written the men a pardon even before the court had reached its decision. In the end they served just 6 months in prison.

Thus, while there existed international condemnation regarding the events that had taken place in the Meiwes case, it proved difficult to differentiate such conduct on either medical or legal grounds. Moreover, in the English case of R. v. *Dudley and Stevens* (1884), not only was it difficult to establish a legal justification for punishing the defendants, but the public actually considered the men as heroes and demanded that they be set free.

What these two cases clearly illustrate is that no matter how abhorrent a particular form of behaviour appears to be, there is nothing about the specific nature of an act itself that makes it inherently 'mad' or 'bad'. In fact, studies that have attempted to empirically establish the existence of universal forms of deviant conduct have also failed (Hagan, 1994; Wilkins, 1964).

Why is the medicalization of criminal behaviour controversial?

Medical ideology and the medicalization of criminal behaviour

In response to earlier comments, practitioners might be prepared to freely acknowledge that there may not currently exist a known organic aetiology or effective treatment for certain forms of criminal behaviour, but that such a fact does not preclude the prospect that one might eventually be found. Nor, they might argue, does the social constructionist conception of deviance devalue the significance of employing a medical ideology. In other words, the medicalization of criminal behaviour provides us with the cognitive tools to be able to make sense of such deviant conduct and manage it in the most humanitarian way possible.

Thus, by defining some types of unacceptable behaviour as an 'illness', independent of any confirmation as to the biological basis of such actions, it becomes possible to offer some help to the individual offender/patient through treatment as well as to satisfy the interests of society to be protected. The following case study serves as a poignant illustration of this point:

CASE STUDY 6

In November 2004 Heather Vinkenbrink, aged 45, was found not guilty by reason of insanity for the murder of her daughter. The jury heard that Mrs Vinkenbrink had become increasingly agitated over the previous few months and believed that her 7-year-old daughter, Lily, was going to be attacked by paedophiles. In an effort to protect Lily from what her mother considered to be an imminent threat, she drowned her in a nearby river, believing that this was the only way to ensure her safety. In what the judge declared to be a 'desperately sad case' both the prosecution and defence accepted the psychiatric testimony that Heather Vinkenbrink was suffering from paranoid schizophrenia. Heather is now receiving treatment within a secure psychiatric facility under the Mental Health Act.

Such tragically 'bad' and 'sad' events can only be meaningfully and satisfactorily dealt with by conceptualizing the offender as in some way 'mad'. Thus, the medical redefinition of Heather's deviant experiences makes it possible for her to be diverted away from the criminal justice system and afforded the status of the 'sick' role (Parsons, 1975), where Heather's problems can be socially controlled, but within regimes that are ideologically therapeutic rather than punitive.

The 'sick' role exempts offender/patients from normal social obligations in terms of blame and responsibility, which often act as barriers to meaningful understanding. For example, traditionally children described in terms of being easily distracted, impulsive and hyperactive would have received punishment for their disobedient and difficult conduct. Today, however, we recognize such behaviour as the classic symptoms of Attention Deficit Hyperactivity Disorder (ADHD) and offer various forms of treatment and support in order to better manage such problems.

However, although at face value it may seem humanitarian to conceptualize criminal behaviour as a form of sickness, there are significant social consequences associated with adopting such an ideological approach.

Medicalization and the depoliticizing of criminal behaviour

The assumption that there exists a biomedical basis to deviant behaviour gives the impression that the decisions made by mental health practitioners about the nature of particular forms of conduct are depoliticized; that judgements are reached within an objective and dispassionate context, detached from moral or social considerations. However, in the absence of an established scientific basis to mental health behavioural classification systems, it is argued that the process of defining actions as either 'mad' or 'bad' is governed by social values, which in turn are intricately linked to the views of the dominant political order within society (Foucault, 1973).

In fact, history tells us that in addition to the criminal law, medicine has developed as a profession of social control; it has evolved as an appendage of the state and is used in order to reinforce the existing political and moral consensus (Szasz, 1970). Moreover, Foucault (1978) has predicted that over time we are likely to see these two social control forces gradually redefine themselves in favour of placing greater emphasis on their similarities rather than their differences. Specifically, Foucault argues that alliances will eventually be created that link psychiatric knowledge with knowledge about criminal justice matters for the purpose of developing new definitions of deviance and devising different forms of social surveillance. Furthermore, it is anticipated that this borderland between mental health and criminological matters is likely to expand its influence and eventually have a fundamental impact on how we politically conceptualize deviant behaviour. In recent years, this transformation and the significance of this borderland has become manifestly apparent, and is evident in at least three ways.

First, what we have experienced in the last few decades is an epistemological shift in our efforts to achieve a sense of ontological security. In other words, we have started to move away from traditional ideological approaches concerned with trying to make the world a 'safer' place through punishing the guilty and treating the sick. Instead, new ways of understanding are being formulated directed towards defining socially deviant conduct not as 'mad' or 'bad', but predominantly in terms of the public and private 'risk of harm' certain actions present, and how this level of risk can best be contained, managed and controlled (Beck, 1992; Feeley and Simon, 1992).

Secondly, towards this new form of practice we are starting to see a greater emphasis on the medicalization and hence control of a wide range of behaviours that have traditionally been managed by defining them as either socially disruptive or morally unacceptable. For example, both the DSM-III and DSM-IV have succeeded in broadening the types of behaviour to be defined as mental disorders to include antisocial personality disorder, ADHD and various substance abuse disorders (Menzies and Webster, 1989). Conversely, society is also starting to witness an expansion in the range of behaviours that have been criminalized. For example, Faulkner (2000) has observed that there currently exist around 8,000 different crimes within Britain and that approximately 140 new crimes are being created each year, a trend which the government anticipates is likely to continue indefinitely (Faulkner, 2000).

Finally, in addition to the emergence of new forms of deviance we are also starting to witness the creation of apparently new forms of knowledge, professionalisms and services which are currently prefixed by the label 'forensic': psychiatry, psychology, nursing, social work, conferences, textbooks, journals, etc. As there has been no recent scientific advancement in our understanding of individuals defined as 'mentally disordered offenders' we can only assume that this army of professionals is being prepared to occupy, colonize and ultimately legitimize the existence of this new medico-legal borderland.

It is also interesting to observe that not only does the net of social control appear to be widening, but there seems to be some evidence to suggest that it is only covering those forms of conduct that the most powerful political and moral entrepreneurs within society deem to be unsuitable (Taylor, Walton and Young, 1973; Becker, 1963). (To illustrate this point see chapter 3 for racial prejudice, chapter 5 for sexuality conceptualized as mental illness and chapter 10 for an overview of the risk agenda in mental health care.)

Today professionals medicalize and/or criminalize what the majority within society apparently consider to be morally dubious practices such as substance abuse (but not alcohol), excessive gambling (but not the national lottery), bigamy (but not adultery), having sexual intercourse with someone under 16 years old, and euthanasia. Indeed, how often are practitioners concerned with questioning the criminality or mental health of individuals responsible for polluting the environment by dumping toxic emissions into our rivers, the manufacture and distribution of products known to be faulty and likely to cause considerable public harm and poor working practices that maim or even kill employees. To emphasize this last situation, read the following case study and bear in mind that the employer only received a fine for his actions.

CASE STUDY 7

In May 1998 one of the 75-foot-long industrial bread ovens owned by a baking company in Leicester, England broke down. Regulations stated that to cool down sufficiently for maintenance work the oven had to be left switched off for 12 hours. However, intent on saving time and money, the employer ignored this guidance and sent two engineers in to fix the problem after just a couple of hours had passed. They travelled along the conveyor used to carry the dough, but while the outside was cool, the centre was still over 100 degrees centigrade. One of the engineers had a radio and tried to relay a panicked message that it was too hot. Unfortunately, the conveyor did not have a reverse function and so there was no way of getting the men out in time. Both men died from heat exhaustion and severe burns.

One can only speculate, but if such an event had taken place outside an economic environment, would the consequences for the offender have been the same? The point is that the implicit assumptions often held concerning the humanitarian and scientific nature of medicine and mental health practice tend to obfuscate the fact that judgements about deviant behaviour and decisions regarding who needs to be socially controlled are not depoliticized; made within a moral or political vacuum. Instead, practitioners are employees of the state and as such are beholden to the decision-making processes of those with the most wealth and power. The fact that there exists a strong interrelationship between political considerations and the medicalization of criminal behaviour will be clearly evident in your own response to the following question: 'As a mental health practitioner, how comfortable would you be working with the definitions of mental disorder and crime used to enforce the moral and political values of the former Nazi regime within Germany, or the conceptualizations of deviance used to uphold the political ideology underlying the former apartheid regime in South Africa?'

Medicalization and the individualised status of criminal offenders

The medicalization of criminal behaviour encourages exploration for the causes of deviance within the individual offender rather than as a result of wider social forces. A potential practical consequence arising from such an approach is that politicians and professionals may become drawn towards simplified policies and solutions for managing unacceptable conduct. After all, it is easier to afford psychiatrists the power to define social problems as the product of some form of 'sickness' than it is for society to confront the real possibility that the complex sociopolitical fabric of our very way of life may actually be flawed. For example, consider the following case study:

CASE STUDY 8

Tom is 11 years old; he is disruptive at school, difficult to manage at home, and has been cautioned several times by the police for public disorder offences. Both the school and Tom's parents have tried a range of punishment and reward schemes to try and modify his behaviour, but nothing seems to work. Everyone is exhausted by the whole experience, and so it is suggested that medical advice be sought. This concludes that since nothing else has worked and the symptoms fit, Tom must have ADHD and medication is prescribed. After a while the child's behaviour seems to change and everyone views this as a medical success.

The difficulty here is that by focusing on Tom's behaviour in terms of symptoms and defining them as a mental health problem, we ignore the possibility that his conduct is in fact not an illness, but a natural response to particular social circumstances. In other words, our attention is diverted away from potential difficulties within the family, school, community and society in general that may be responsible for generating such conduct, towards pathologizing the individual (Laing, 1961, 1967). In these terms it almost seems acceptable that some people should live with social disadvantages such as poverty, poor quality housing, a disruptive family environment and inadequate learning experiences. The difficulty only arises when they start to react to those disadvantages.

Thus, a significant implication arising from medicalizing some forms of criminality is that it redefines understanding of social problems. The moment deviant behaviour is defined as a medical phenomenon it becomes inaccessible to the general public because it can no longer be made sense of as a rational (albeit unacceptable) response to social circumstances. Instead, it is conceptualized in terms of predominantly internal causal forces that do not seem to relate at all to everyday experiences.

As a consequence, the individual becomes the 'property' of experts who by virtue of their training in the use of scientific/medical research and knowledge apparently possess a specialized understanding of such deviants. After all, mentally disordered offenders, so the public is led to believe, constitute a biologically different group of people to ourselves and that is why we need practitioners with particular knowledge, skills and status in order to deal with their difficulties. Actually, the individualization of social problems gives rise to a rather interesting pattern of circular reasoning which self-perpetuates the need for professionals: first, mental health practitioners create the problem by suggesting (but not proving) that some forms of deviant conduct can be medically explained, and then purport to be able to resolve the problem that it has created in the first place. If the logic of this argument is extended a little further, it could be claimed that mental health practitioners are in fact the root cause of mental disorders. Moreover, pushing this pattern of reasoning a little more shows that, despite there being no pathological basis to deviant conduct, biomedically orientated practitioners still insist on trying to persuade society that it really exists, which according to their own classification systems constitutes delusional behaviour!

Of course, this is not to support the contention that all mental health practitioners are psychologically disturbed. In fact, what is being highlighted here is operating at the metaphysical level of analysis; playing with reason and logic in order to exploit flaws implicit within our taken-for-granted way of doing things. This is not to deny the reality of the suffering and difficulties individuals sometimes find themselves in. Nor is it our intention to suggest that the medical ideology has not had a significant beneficial impact on many people's lives. Instead, a metaphysical approach allows us to 'step outside the box' and take the time to question the currently dominant role of medicine within mental health practice. In particular, to claim exclusive access to knowledge about certain types of deviant behaviour ensures that the general public remains subservient to privileged groups of professionals. This is problematic because it locates too much power and control with 'experts' who are afforded a considerable amount of unfettered authority to make a series of fundamental decisions about our lives in terms of a whole range of issues such as who should be punished, treated, rehabilitated, detained or declared as a risk to society. By making such a claim we imply no malevolence on the part of mental health practitioners, but are simply raising the possibility that the road of good intentions is often paved with unintended consequences.

For example, diverting mentally disordered offenders away from the criminal justice system and into mental health care clearly has several advantages for the offender/patient. However, by affording individuals the status of the 'sick' role and putting professionals in charge can also cause significant confusion and ambiguity about where responsibility for the criminal conduct should lie. The interpretation of events in terms of apportioning blame, praise or responsibility is an important social process (Lerner, 1980). By suspending the question of culpability, diverted offender/patients are left open to abuse as their social status becomes undefined; in effect, they have no status and become beholden to those who are deemed to be responsible for their actions (Parsons, 1975). Under such circumstances, there exists the real danger that mentally disordered offenders become dehumanized; treated as dysfunctional objects that can be measured, analysed and probed all in the name of science and the protection of the public. Moreover, such an unfettered invasion of the human system can lead, and indeed has, led to the development of some staggeringly degrading and unethical practices (Foucault, 1973; Szasz, 1961).

Furthermore, the medicalization of criminal behaviour also tends to play down the potential significance of the classicist notion of free will. In turn, this surrounds individual offenders with an excusing culture, which makes it easy and indeed acceptable for them to consider themselves as sick or dysfunctional in some way (Parsons, 1975). The risk here is that the sick role status may give offenders the impression that they should be absolved of all responsibility for their conduct, that their actions are beyond their control and that they need not feel under any moral obligation to attempt to change.

Can 'mentally disordered offenders' ever be viewed as a normal and beneficial aspect of society?

Understanding mentally disordered offenders from a social constructionist approach also raises the possibility that categorizing some people in this way could actually constitute a normal and beneficial aspect of our lives. Imagine for a moment living in a society where no 'madness' or 'badness' exists, a society or indeed a world in which there are no forms of 'crazy', bizarre' 'odd', 'strange' or 'unusual' behaviour, no multiple murders, sex offenders, arsonists, street robbers, burglars, vandals or thieves. In fact, a social utopia in which deviant conduct of any kind simply does not exist.

Well, according to the influential French sociologist Émile Durkheim (1858–1917) such a world is difficult to imagine because mental disorder and crime are in fact normal, natural and therefore an essential part of human existence. He goes on to argue that there is nothing unusual about the existence of mentally disordered offenders; they have always existed and are found in all societies. More specifically Durkheim qualifies his remarks by suggesting that deviance, however we wish to define it, is socially functional in the sense that it serves a number of important roles within society (Durkheim, 1982).

First, Durkheim argues that the only way society could ever rid itself of mental disorder and crime is if there existed social homogeneity. However, because people are naturally inclined towards acting and thinking differently from one another, some people, while trying to meet their own needs, will inevitably behave in ways that others will view as deviant. Even if there did exist a biological basis to mental disorder and we could in fact find universal forms of conduct that everyone agreed constitute crimes, their eradication would make little difference because the very existence of human diversity would ensure the perpetuation of deviance. In other words, any differences, regardless of how minor they may appear to be, such as having tattoos, wearing clothes with hoods, speaking too loudly on a mobile phone, believing in horoscopes or smoking in public buildings will inevitably be elevated to the status of 'mental disorders' and/or 'crimes'.

In fact, Durkheim argues that our preoccupation with classifying and labelling behaviour is such a fundamental condition of social life that it actually stops us from going insane! His reasoning is that the only way to completely rid ourselves of mentally disordered and criminal deviants would be to become pathologically obsessed with seeking out and destroying human variations, a trend which must logically continue until eventually we all think and act in exactly the same way.

Secondly, Durkheim suggests that social constructions of mental disorder and crime may be directly beneficial to society as the actual process of labelling deviant behaviour helps society shape and define the status of existing moral boundaries. In other words, by pathologizing or criminalizing certain forms of conduct, society is in effect drawing lines in the sand between sane/insane and good/bad, and then inadvertently challenging society to debate the relative status of this line. For example, at the present time the moral, medical and legal status of cannabis is highly contested; on one level its reclassification as a class C drug under the Misuse of Drugs Act (1971) suggests support for making it legal to possess cannabis for personal use. On another level, some practitioners within the medical profession have raised concerns about its impact on people's mental health, while others have supported its therapeutic aspects. On yet another level, campaigners argue that it should retain its moral and legal status as a socially unacceptable and unlawful substance. Without establishing behavioural boundaries in the first place we would have nothing to challenge.

Actually, the very notion that we have dynamic moral boundaries as to what should be deemed acceptable and unacceptable conduct gives rise to a number of intriguing contradictions that clearly demonstrate the social construction of all forms of deviance. For example, the DSM-IV now recognizes alcoholism as a disease, which can be associated with severe mental health problems; research also suggests a link between alcohol consumption and certain types of crime. Yet despite the fact that it causes so much social harm, our solution has been to make alcohol more readily available to the public through longer licensing hours. The point being made and emphasized here is not that relaxation of criminal laws in relation to certain drugs and alcohol is necessarily wrong, but that the way we define and deal with notions of deviance are far more complex and subtle than could be tolerated within a purely scientific/medical conceptualization of social problems.

Finally, mental disorder and crime may also be viewed as beneficial to the extent that such notions help direct our attention towards problems within society that otherwise may not be immediately obvious. For example, if rates of either 'crazy behaviour' and/or 'criminal behaviour' become too high this may signal the presence of social problems, which in turn might activate the development of new policy initiatives in order to make improvements in areas such as housing, job opportunities, community care or surveillance.

Conversely, if such definitions of deviance did not exist then this would lead to the implicit assumption that all was well with the world. Thus, the social value in being able to categorize certain behaviours as either 'mad' or 'bad' makes it possible for society to recognize and express its concerns about such issues. For example, if forms of conduct such as: paranoia, obsessiveness, extreme sadness, homelessness, child abuse, domestic violence and environmental pollution were not declared as deviant then they could continue to take place as legitimized forms of conduct because they would have failed to provoke any public reaction.

Conclusion

A social constructionist perspective of mental disorder and crime helps us to reconceptualize a range of issues often overlooked during the course of daily practice. It is hoped that the critical comments expressed in this chapter help to challenge some of the commonly held assumptions about 'madness' and 'badness'. It is too simplistic to think that these forms of deviance constitute a stain on the fabric of society which once understood can be safely removed either through medication and/or incarceration. Instead, while some forms of deviant conduct may represent individual and personal tragedy, they may also be interpreted as a necessary and essential feature of the way in which one makes sense of the world.

Ultimately, the message for mental health practitioners is straightforward; the real significance of the medical ideology will only be realized once notions of mental disorder and crime are conceptualized as intricately bound to the political, social and cultural context in which these deviant actions take place.

EDITORS' QUESTIONS

Issues of difference

- When does sexual expression become a crime?
- Are there age-related crimes?
- How do different cultures consider and deal with crime?

Relevance to practice

- How do mental health professionals assess insight and remorse?
- In what way can professional disciplines improve liaison within the justice system?
- In what ways do your beliefs about acceptable conduct influence your practice?

Investigate

- How is a forensic history assessed in your service or practice?
- What is the social constructionist perspective of mental disorder and crime?
- What are the treatment options within forensic mental health services?

Suggested further reading

Downes, D. and Rock, P. (2003) *Understanding Deviance* (4th edn). Oxford: Oxford University Press.

Williams, K. (2004) *Criminology*. Oxford: Oxford University Press.

References

APA (2000) *The Diagnostic and Statistical Manual of Mental Disorders (4th edn, Text Revision DSM-TR)*. Washington, DC: American Psychiatric Association.

Beck, U. (1992) *Risk Society: Towards a New Modernity*. London: Sage.

Becker, H. (1963) *Outsiders*. New York: The Free Press.

Clark, L.A., Watson, D. and Reynolds, S. (1995) Diagnosis and classification of psychopathology: challenges to the current system and future directions. *Annual Review of Psychology* 46: 121–53.

Colombo, A. (1997) *Understanding Mentally Disorder Offenders: A Multi-agency Perspective*. London: Ashgate.

Colombo, A., Bendelow, G., Fulford, W.K.M. and Williams, S. (2003) Evaluating the influence of implicit models of mental disorder on processes of shared decision making within community-based multi-disciplinary teams. *International Journal of Social Science and Medicine* 56: 1557–70.

Criminal Justice Act (1991) Schedule 1: www.opsi.gov.uk/acts/acts1991/Ukpga_19910053_en_1.htm [Accessed 01/02/08]

Criminal Procedure (Insanity and Unfitness to Plead) Act (1991) www.opsi.gov.uk/ACTS/acts1991/ukpga_19910025_en_1 [Accessed: 01/02/08].

Descartes, R. (1997) *Key Philosophical Writings*. Ware: Wordsworth.

Downes, D. and Rock, P. (2003) *Understanding Deviance*. (4th edn). Oxford: Oxford University Press.

Durkheim, E. (1982) *Rules of the Sociological Method*. New York: The Free Press.

Ellis, L. (1996) A discipline in peril: sociology's future hinges on curing biophobia. *American Sociologist* 27: 21–41.

Faulkner, D. (2000) *Crime, State and Citizen*. Winchester: Waterside Press.

Feeley, M.M. and Simon, J (1992) The new penology: notes on the emerging strategy of corrections and its implications. *Criminology* 30(4): 452–74.

Foucault, M. (1973) *The Birth of the Clinic*. New York: Vintage Books.

Foucault, M. (1978) *Discipline and Punish*. New York Vintage Books.

Gottfredson, M.R. and Hirschi, T. (1990) *A General Theory of Crime*. Stanford, CA: Stanford University Press.

Hagan, J. (1994) *Crime and Disrepute*. Thousand Oaks C.A: Pine Forge Press.

Halfpenny, P. (1982) *Positivism and Sociology: Explaining Social Life*. London: Allen & Unwin.

Home Office (1990) *Circular 66/90. Provision for Mentally Disordered Offenders*. London: HMSO.

Infanticide Act (1938) www.statutelaw.gov.uk/content.aspx?LegType=All+Primary&PageNumber=80&NavFrom=2&parentActiveTextDocId=1085464&activetextdocid=1085467 [Accessed 01/02/08]

Laing, R.D. (1961) *The Self and Others*. London: Tavistock.

Laing, R.D. (1967) *The Politics of Experience*. Harmondsworth: Penguin.

Lamb, Lady Caroline (1812) Writing in her journal after having met Byron. Referred to in Prins, H. (2005) Mental disorder and violent crime: a problematic relationship. *Probation Journal* 52(4): 333–57.

Lerner, M. (1980) *The Belief in a Just World: A Fundamental Delusion*. New York: Plenum Press.

Lishman, W.A. (1997) *Organic Psychiatry*. (3rd edn). Oxford: Blackwell.

McKenna, P.J. (1997) *Schizophrenia and Related Syndromes*. Hove: Psychology Press.

McNaughton Rules (1843) Case 8 Eng. Rep. 718.

Mental Health Act (1983) London: HMSO.

Menzies, R.J. and Webster, C.D. (1989) Mental disorder and violent crime. In N. Weiner and M.E. Wolfgang (eds) *Pathways to Criminal Violence*. Newbury Park, CA: Sage.

Mickalowski, R. (1985) *Order, Law and Crime*. New York: Random House.

Misuse of Drugs Act (1971) London: HMSO.

Murray, R., Walsh, E. and Arsenault, L. (2002) Some possible answers to questions about schizophrenia that have concerned John Gunn. *Criminal Behaviour and Mental Health* Supplement **12**: S4–9.

Niehoff, D. (1999) *The Biology of Violence*. New York: Free Press.

Ormerod, D. (2005) *Smith and Hogan: Criminal Law*. Oxford: Oxford University Press.

Parsons, T. (1975) The sick role and the role of the physician reconsidered. *Milbank Memorial Fund Quarterly. Health and Society* **53**(3): 257–78.

Pilgrim, D. and Rogers, A. (1999) *A Sociology of Mental Health and Illness*. Buckingham: Open University Press.

Reed Report (1992) *Report into Mentally Disordered Offenders. and Others Who Require Similar Services*. CM2088. London: HMSO.

Ritchie, J.H., Dick, D. and Lingham, R. (1994) *The Report of the Inquiry into the Care and Treatment of Christopher Clunis*. London: HMSO.

Schwartz, S. (1999) Biological approaches to psychiatric disorders. In A.V. Horwitz and T.L. Scheid (eds) *A Handbook for the Study of Mental Health*. Cambridge: Cambridge University Press.

Sellin, T. (1938) *Culture Conflict and Crime*. New York: Social Science Research Council.

Sexual Offences Act (1967) London: Stationery Office.

Sexual Offences (Amendment) Act (2000) www.opsi.gov.uk/acts/acts2000/ukpga_20000044_en_1.htm [Accessed 01/02/08].

Sexual Offences Act 2003 (Commencement) (Scotland) (2004) Edinburgh: Scottish Government.

Suicide Act (1961) http://www.opsi.gov.uk/RevisedStatutes/Acts/ukpga/1961/cukpga_19610060_en_1 [accessed 01/02/08].

Sutherland, E. and Cressey, D. (1970) *Principles of Criminology*. (6th edn). Philadelphia: Lippincott.

Szasz, T. (1961) *The Myth of Mental Illness*. New York: Dell.

Szasz, T. (1970) *The Manufacture of Madness*. New York: Dell.

Taylor, I., Walton, P. and Young, J. (1973) *The New Criminology*. London: Routledge.

Timmermans, S. and Gabe, J. (2004) *Partners in Health, Partners in Crime*. Oxford: Blackwell.

Wakefield, J.C. (1992) Disorder as a harmful dysfunction: a conceptual critique of DSM-IIIR's definition of mental disorder. *Psychological Review* **99**: 232–47.

Wilkins, L. (1964) *Social Deviance*. London: Tavistock.

Williams, K. (2004) *Criminology*. Oxford: Oxford University Press.

Wilson, E.O. (1975) *Sociobiology: The New Synthesis*. Cambridge, MA: Harvard University Press.

WHO (1992) *The ICD 10 – The International Classification of Mental and Behavioural Disorders: Clinical Descriptions and Diagnostic Guidelines*. Geneva: World Health Organization.

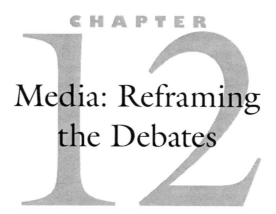

Media: Reframing the Debates

Lesley Henderson

BRIEF CHAPTER OUTLINE

This chapter sets out to reframe the debate on media and mental distress and explore different media formats. TV news and press coverage is the first area tackled, detailing such concerns as playing on public fears through sensationalized headlines that isolate mental illness specifically. The section is navigated through an exploration of performance and authenticity in both documentary and reality television. The author highlights how newer formats play on old stereotypes of mental illness to increase viewer ratings. The next consideration examines television drama, from ER to EastEnders. Finally, the impact of media on audiences shows how the public draw images from both factual and fictional media interchangeably. The chapter ends with a look towards more balanced representations.

Introduction

This chapter critically examines some of the central debates concerning media and mental distress. Numerous studies have made connections between media coverage and public beliefs about mental health and the negative coverage of mental health issues is considered to bear significant responsibility for fuelling public prejudice and misconceptions. The stereotyping and limited range of portrayals of service users are believed to dissuade those in distress from seeking help or to mask their symptoms through substance abuse. Conditions such as schizophrenia have been associated with particular stigma, and the media stereotyping of those affected by such diagnoses is considered to have significant repercussions for their families, carers and other members of their social network. Such negative reporting is considered to play a role in policy decision-making, and to both increase restrictive care and surveillance and at the same time to undermine initiatives which aim to support service users living in the community. In light of reforms to mental health-care systems in Britain and the rest of Europe, the reporting of violent incidents involving those with mental illness is considered to play a role in creating a professional preoccupation with risk and dangerousness. Such reforms are regarded as having a disproportionate focus on compulsory treatment and detention, with serious repercussions for the rights of users of services (Brindle, 2006) (see also mind.org.uk and communitycare.org.uk).

In general, positive liaison with the mass media is now regarded as providing the cornerstone of any successful health campaign. Yet the profile of media reporting concerning mental distress has proved surprisingly resistant to change. This is despite the fact that a number of organizations now proactively promote the perspectives of service users in the mass media (Harper, 2005: 462; Plumb, 1993). Media strategies such as World Mental Health Day (10 October) are designed to focus media coverage positively and such initiatives borrow from campaigning in other areas of health and illness such as HIV and AIDS and breast cancer. Mental Health Media Awards represent a move away from media 'blame' and instead reward more positive and challenging representations. Despite these initiatives the consistent and frequent portrayal in the media of those in mental distress as dangerous, volatile and a threat to others suggests that this group remains excluded as media sources. This absence it is argued undermines initiatives, which seek to present service users as active citizens. Clearly this is not a new problem – mental illness and prejudice have a trajectory, which predates modern media and is deeply ingrained culturally (Signorielli, 1993).

At the same time it is important that we recognize that the mass media is not homogeneous and diverse media formats are produced in different ways and with different target audiences in mind. It is an oversimplification to suggest that individual media professionals would wish to promote misleading images of those in mental distress. However, as discussed later, the media values and commercial imperatives, which underpin how newspapers and television formats are produced, may limit the range of representations which results. It is also worth noting that there is no simple single message which every affected person would wish to be promoted in the media. Nonetheless these negative and systematic patterns of coverage deserve to be explained. Mental distress, particularly acute conditions such as schizophrenia, are, in media accounts, commonly linked to violent crime. This is surprisingly consistent, across format (from television news to entertainment) and geography (UK, US and European media).

Media coverage is considered to play a significant role in fuelling public prejudice and contributing to stigmatization (Philo, 1996; Wahl, 1995). A study found that when the general public were asked about appropriate treatment for schizophrenia as many as 95 per cent agreed with enforced treatment. This has been taken as evidence that perceptions of danger perpetuated by media reporting have a role to play in creating cultural acceptance of coerced treatment (Wahl, 2003: 1596). Images of the mentally ill in other media formats such as children's cartoons and films have been identified as mainly negative, depicting those with psychiatric disorders as unattractive, violent and criminal (Wahl, 2003).

This chapter highlights some of the complexity of the debates concerning media and mental health. It broadly addresses the following questions: What is the nature of coverage? To what extent is this the case across different media formats? What are the international dimensions to the problem? What role do media practitioners play in developing such negative coverage? What effects might these images have on audiences? The chapter is structured to explore different media formats in order to draw out the differences and commonalities across genre and, where possible, to also examine the perspectives of those involved in creating them.

The overall aim here is to address the possibilities and constraints of different media formats for providing more balanced accounts of mental health. In so doing a number of UK and international cases will be identified to highlight key findings and to engage with debates concerning media values and the broad topic of mental health from within sociology and communications as well as public health/health promotion models.

Icons of public disorder: TV news and press coverage

A large number of studies have explored how mental distress is represented in television news and newspapers. In the wake of the move from institutionalized care in psychiatric hospitals towards a policy of 'care in the community', during the mid-1990s a wide-ranging UK study was undertaken of the reporting of mental health in the mass media (Philo, 1996; Philo, Henderson and McLaughlin, 1993).

Although criticized for over-generalizing across media formats, this study is considered to be groundbreaking in its scope (Harper, 2005). It was designed to address how mental health issues were framed in the factual media (press and television news, current affairs programmes) as well as other media formats (soap opera, comedy, children's television) which have traditionally been overlooked in analyses of health and media. The study also made important links between the nature of media coverage, production processes and public beliefs about mental distress. These points will be explored later. In this section some of the key findings from the study of press and television news are highlighted and examined as to how they relate to other work concerned with possible links between factual news media reporting and policy decision-making.

The most striking finding of the Glasgow Media Group study was the high prevalence of media stories in which those referenced as 'mentally ill' were associated with the theme of 'violence to others'. Indeed, across the sample as a whole, a total of 66 per cent of all items which referenced mental health were in relation to 'harm to others', and a minority depicted 'self-harm' (13 per cent of all items) (Philo, 1996). Thus during the sampling period there were numerous reports of attacks on strangers in which the protagonist was labelled 'maniac', 'madman' and 'psycho' (Philo, 1996: 50–64).

One particular story involving an alleged random attack on a young boy received high-profile media treatment. Various reports described how a 'lunatic' had poured petrol on a 7-year-old child and set fire to his face. This story was reported extensively and featured in lurid front-page headlines in the popular tabloid newspaper the *Daily Mirror*: 'Set on fire by a maniac'. Other newspapers reported that police were seeking a 'maniac' (*Sun*) or a 'fiend' (*Daily Star*) in connection with the incident. Yet when it emerged later that the boys had been playing with a petrol can and had in fact invented the story of a mythical 'lunatic' as a cover story, the *Daily Mirror* buried their retraction of the report on page 13, whereas other papers neglected to retract the story.

During the same period there was a wave of news stories concerning 'crazed fans' stalking various celebrities (pop stars, models and sports figures). Typical headlines included 'Psycho fan stalks Cindy' (*Daily Sport*). When the tennis player Monica Seles was stabbed during a tennis match this provoked widespread reporting in which the attacker was described as a 'nutter' (*Daily Star*), a 'madman' (*Daily Sport*) and a 'maniac' (*Daily Mirror*). These stories linking mental illness and violent crime did not only appear more frequently than any other story theme, but these stories were more likely to enjoy a high media prominence, appearing in front-page or headline stories, whereas other more sympathetic items appeared in less prominent positions, including the problem pages of magazines (Philo and Secker, 1999).

Occasionally the protagonists of such 'random' incidents themselves become publicly known. A study of UK press reporting of two cases involving people with a diagnosis of schizophrenia revealed that emotive and lurid headlines are not simply the province of the 'tabloid' media. The cases involved Christopher Clunis, who killed a stranger (Jonathan Zito) at a London Underground station and Ben Silcock, who was mauled when he climbed into the lion's den at London Zoo. These cases attracted familiar headline-catching language, but significantly the interest was largely in the 'quality' rather than 'tabloid' press (Hallam, 2002). Indeed, at least initially, there was surprisingly little press interest in the death of Jonathan Zito (a young man randomly killed in a public place). This dearth of interest changed when it became apparent, during the court trial some months later, that Clunis had been diagnosed with schizophrenia.

Hallam argues that this trajectory suggests that even random, violent incidents are not in themselves newsworthy but, as she describes, 'it is the mental illness of the perpetrator that tips the scales' (Hallam 2002: 29–30). Both of these cases formed the basis for campaigns which lobbied for improved treatment. The journalist Marjorie Wallace, a mental health campaigner and Chief Executive of SANE, also happened to be a friend of Silcock's father. She used the case as a platform to write personalized and emotive accounts of the background to the incident. Wallace explained in an article in the *Daily Mail* why Ben Silcock had undertaken this apparently irrational and dangerous act – the answer, she wrote, 'in one shuddering word, is schizophrenia' (Hallam, 2002: 29). Indeed, Wallace was contacted by then government Health Minister, Virginia Bottomley, who promised a 'shake-up of mental health laws' in response to Silcock's 'schizophrenia torment'.

While the Zito Trust (set up in the name of Jonathan Zito, who was killed by Christopher Clunis) and those associated with the Silcock case were lobbying for improved provision for people in crisis, the publication of the Ten Point Plan which followed in the wake of these incidents focused instead on a scheme for supervised discharge of psychiatric patients considered at risk, and registers of mentally ill people discharged to live in their own home (DH, 1993). Hallam argues that the focus of media coverage means that 'the public could reasonably assume that all tragedies could be averted if people with a diagnosis of schizophrenia took their medication and complied with treatment' (Hallam, 2002: 32). Regardless of the intentions of campaigners, by highlighting killings by those with mental illness media reporting is considered to fuel public fear and to help create a climate in which restrictive care is deemed necessary to contain public fear.

Around the same time, the Boyd Report (DH, 1994) published a preliminary confidential inquiry into suicides and homicides by people with mental illness. It had been set up following a small number of high-profile cases in which those who had been diagnosed as mentally ill had killed themselves or others. The main findings challenged many of the myths in circulation. The report emphasized that the victims of those who had used psychiatric services were known to them (thus challenging the 'stranger–danger' theme promoted in many media accounts) and that most perpetrators had been seen by medical professionals in the 24 hours before the attack, with most (three quarters of those people who killed) complying with prescribed medication.

However despite this, the media reporting consisted largely of newspaper and television headlines which played on public fears of stranger attack by 'schizophrenics' defaulting on their medication (Crepaz-Keay, 1996: 38). Typical headlines included: 'One murder a fortnight by mentally ill' (*Daily Telegraph*); 'Scandal of loonies freed to kill' (*Daily Star*) and 'Sick and dangerous' (*Daily Mail*). BBC and independent television reporting was similarly distorted and indeed, at times, also factually incorrect. A BBC report announced that 'many had failed to take prescribed medication' and focused on the case of a man diagnosed with schizophrenia who had killed an occupational therapist (BBC *Nine O'Clock News*).

Yet as Crepaz-Keay points out, this man was receiving depot (injected) medicine and had not in fact defaulted on his medication. Cases such as this are reported in the context of 'psycho-killer on the loose', a theme which is now part of popular cultural mythology. While Crepaz-Keay does not seek to excuse the tragedy of homicides perpetrated by people who had used psychiatric services for all involved, he does argue that on this occasion all sections of the media missed a rare and important opportunity to critique the false perceptions of a link between a diagnosis of mental illness and violence for the sake of a story. As he concludes:

> infrequent and isolated events should not be used by all sections of the media to damn an entire group of people. The deaths were in fact a very small proportion of homicides as a whole, and those who killed were a tiny proportion of those who are mentally distressed. The deaths could not be attributed to a policy of 'releasing' into the community large numbers of 'dangerous' people who refused to take their medication and killed at random.
>
> (Crepaz-Keay, 1996: 43)

In the USA, the names John Hinckley Jr., who attempted to assassinate President Ronald Reagan in 1981 and Andrew Goldstein, dubbed 'the subway psycho' for pushing Kendra Webdale on to the New York City subway tracks in 1999 (leading to 'Kendra's Law') are also believed to have become icons of public fear, symbolizing the failings of the legal and mental health-care systems (Wahl, 2003). We have witnessed similar debates more recently, sparked by the murder of Swedish Foreign Minister, Anna Lindh, on 10 September 2003. Even as the Swedish media reported that there was as yet no suspect in connection with the killing, newspapers were reporting that the police commissioner 'believes that the killer is in the police files and that he can be mentally ill' (*Dagens Nyheter*). A study of press and television reports in the Swedish media found that this reporting assumed that psychological problems are represented as a direct cause of violent crime. This signifies that 'The individual in question *is* his or her mental illness or disorder, and the mental problems mean the person has a predisposition, a tendency to commit violent crimes' (Rassmusen and Hoijer, 2005: 6).

When a 5-year-old girl was murdered in Arvika, Sweden, two days later, the media were swift to proclaim that the attacker had been 'inspired' by Lindh's murder. News reports highlighted that the perpetrator was undergoing voluntary treatment at Arvika's Hospital's psychiatric clinic at the time – he had been told about Anna Lindh's death and 'shortly thereafter he set off for Gategarden where he attacked the girl' (*Dagens Nyheter*). The incident was seen to be indicative of a public culture of great uncertainty. At the time heated debates about the European Monetary Union were ongoing in the Swedish media and politicians were reportedly concerned about the impact of this on mentally ill people as it was believed to make them agitated and confused ('Politicians concerned about the mentally ill'; *Dagens Nyheter*). Partly the problem lies in the assumptions made by the news media – in the case of the man who killed the child it was reported commonly that the perpetrator was 'controlled by voices' and ought to have been placed in compulsory institutional care. In other words, the implication is that 'anyone who hears voices is dangerous – mental illness predisposes to violence' (Rassmusen and Hoijer, 2005: 6).

As touched on earlier, the events which become 'news' are not self-evident but depend on a number of factors that make them 'newsworthy' (Galtung and Ruge, 1965; Ericson, Baraneck and Chan, 1987). The stories discussed above involve violence and crime in connection with mental illness. They encapsulate key criteria and decontextualize events, as Aldridge explains: 'immediacy plus drama plus simplification produces an emphasis on events and persons rather than structures and processes' (Aldridge, 1994: 21). It is known that news media are overly focused on sensational stories in other areas of health and illness (for a discussion see Seale, 2002). Indeed, according to some, '*every* social group is likely to be overrepresented as violent in western news media (and in many other forms of media) (Harper, 2005: 470). Yet the central focus of the studies discussed above points to the very limited set of representations related to those in mental distress, as unpredictable, harmful and to be feared. Such images are believed to fuel public fears of those who are mentally ill and to help create a climate in which there is high public tolerance of compulsory treatment. Such reporting helps to emphasize links between mental illness and dangerousness, and the focus on crime is considered not just to be unhelpful but to compromise journalistic responsibilities of bias and balance – given that a small minority of mental health service users are involved in such acts yet are mainly represented in connection with such crimes (Wahl, 2003).

So why do journalists continue to report the issue in such an 'unbalanced' way? It would be incorrect to assume that individual journalists have a desire to represent mental distress in deliberately skewed ways. The UK journalist David Brindle has reported on mental health and social policy over a number of years and is currently Public Services Editor at the *Guardian* newspaper. He was voted Mental Health Journalist of the Year in 1996 and has often spoken publicly of the complexity which lies behind the news-making process. This is not a preordained process, but rather is often the result of an implicit 'news sense' that addresses the ethos of the newspaper and assumed audience. Sometimes they misjudge public feeling. When the British ex-boxer Frank Bruno was admitted to a mental hospital the *Sun* newspaper had as its front-page headline 'Bonkers Bruno Locked Up' (23 September 2003). The report generated outrage and the readership threatened to boycott the newspaper. It is unclear if this was changing public opinion or public empathy. Brindle describes the process: 'By and large, though, journalists take on-the-run decisions about what to cover, and what not, on the basis not of any written or even verbal guidelines but according to an almost intuitive sense of what fits the bill for the paper in question' (Brindle, 1999: 40).

This 'intuitive' sense of what will work in terms of media formats is not confined to newspaper reporting but permeates and guides media professionals in other areas. Another issue here is that the perspective of people with mental illness is very rarely included. Indeed, very few non-medical experts are invited to act as news sources (Wahl, Wood and Richards, 2002). Again it is important to note that this problem about inequities of access and representation in the media is not confined to the field of mental health but also extends to other disempowered or minority groups. However, if public perceptions of people who have experienced mental distress are to change positively, it seems crucial that individuals are allowed the space and time to speak for themselves. David Crepaz-Keay, Deputy Director of Mental Health Media, has discussed the problem of what he terms the 'missing voice' in mental health representations.

Survivor organizations frequently lack the resources of the large-scale mental health 'official' bodies and often find it difficult to identify survivors willing to act as media sources at short notice.

As Crepaz-Keay comments:

> It's more difficult to get a quick survivor response. It is easy to talk to the Royal College of Psychiatrists', Sane's or Minds's press office who can have someone on *Newsnight* within a few hours' notice. While other people continue to speak on our behalf, the perception of people as patient continues. Just because it's hard work, doesn't mean you shouldn't.
>
> (quoted in Henderson 2007: 119)

The BBC has agreed that wherever possible the service user's voice should be included and that journalists will receive training on reporting disability issues. Clearly there are spaces where survivors may gain access to the media. New more radical factual formats such as *Video Diaries* mark a deliberate attempt by the BBC to allow those disenfranchised in the wider media to present their views (Cross, 2004). The next section of this chapter turns to documentary and reality television formats and how these may provide different spaces for alternative views.

Performance and authenticity: documentary and reality television

The documentary format is assumed to offer significant opportunities for more positive representations and is considered to represent an important public service sphere (Corner 1986; Winston, 1995). Stephen Cross (2004) analyses the possibilities for alternative documentary spaces in three contrasting forms of British current affairs television. Programmes like 'Whose Mind is it Anyway?' *Panorama*; 'A Place of Safety', *Disguises* and 'Mad, Bad or Sad? *Video Diaries*' deal with similar material – the implication of releasing 'mental patients' into the community. Each of these programmes draws on the topic of schizophrenia to discuss the issue. Cross is interested in addressing how television programmes depict schizophrenia visually, in other words, how an unobservable phenomenon is visualized 'such that viewers can recognize that schizophrenia is what is being portrayed' (Cross, 2004: 205). Viewers are provided with a number of visual cues. In the *Panorama* programme the voice-over discusses community supervision orders (CSOs) to control 'mental patients' who refuse medication. It reveals that 'only those regarded as a threat to themselves or others would have Orders imposed', as a close-up of a man playing pool hones in on his dishevelled appearance and facial expression.

Later the programme uses footage from a CSO scheme in the city of Madison, USA, to describe a man being arrested by the police as a 'chronic schizophrenic'. He has been brandishing a knife in a restaurant and the implication is that he has defaulted on his medication. In other words, the police action means that a human tragedy has been narrowly averted. Cross argues that scenes which focus on the man apparently talking to himself in the back of the police car, the retrieved knife on the dashboard and the flashing police siren signify imminent danger. Thus the man is 'transformed into a potentially homicidal schizophrenic whose unobservable violent intentions are rendered graphically observable in the image of the knife' (Cross, 2004: 207).

In the *Disguises* programme a reporter impersonates a 'homeless schizophrenic' to assess the adequacy of care in the community. Using hidden cameras, the reporter adopts strange behaviour designed to attract public attention: lying down in the street and shouting at imagined voices with the aim of being 'sectioned' by the police under the Mental Health Act. However, in practice, his behaviour elicits very little attention – although removing his clothes publicly does result in the police being called, they simply send him away and are unsympathetic to his claims that he hears voices. The programme message is that care in the community does not work: 'It is here that the failure of community care is rendered alarmingly visible in the image of a "mad" and potentially dangerous schizophrenic left to wander unsupervised' (Cross, 2004: 209).

In the *Video Diaries* programme, viewers are presented with a different account of schizophrenia from the perspective of a young woman, 'Sharon'. Her problems are considered to stem from the trauma of her adoption and from the outset the programme positions the 'mentally ill presenter' in different potentially more challenging ways. Thus Sharon introduces her diary to viewers thus: 'You probably don't think you'll crack up. The chances are you might, then you'd be a nutter like me. A doctor will give you a label that sticks to you for the rest of your life. Mine was schizophrenic. Making this diary was hard sharing all my secrets but I really want you to see me, the person I am behind the label' (Cross, 2004: 210).

Cross argues that such an address to viewers (using traditionally pejorative terms like 'nutter') acts to highlight Sharon's own ambivalence (concerning 'difference' and 'sameness') which are rarely visible in traditional media accounts. While each of these programmes confirms that 'schizophrenics' are seen as 'identifiably' different, these visual representations have important implications for challenging social exclusion, 'visual images representing them as though they belong elsewhere are manifestly unhelpful' (Cross, 2004: 212).

As with many of the studies outlined here we know very little about how audiences may respond – it is important not to assume that the impact of these programmes can be inferred from academic analysis of programme content. Far less is known about how these programmes are produced and so the perspectives of documentary makers will now be explored (Henderson, 1996, 2007: ch. 6).

Despite common assumptions that documentary producers have more autonomy than other media professionals, in practice there are a number of key constraints which have serious implications for how this format portrays mental illness. Central constraints come from limited budgets and demand for audience-pleasing television, simply termed 'good television'. Strongly held beliefs about 'what audiences want' of course plays a central role in how material is selected and presented. Filming and editing are governed by factors of narrative pace and drama, qualities that are mistakenly assumed to be the sole remit of drama programming. Thus documentary film series involve casting decisions (which 'patients' will be selected for filming? How will their story be told?). Producers must construct a strong gripping narrative regardless of the 'reality' of the circumstances they are filming. As one producer who filmed in a psychiatric institution explained:

> There are two stages I think where what is needed as a programme-maker conflicts with basically what is there – one is in the filming of it and another is in the editing. You are looking for some drama. You know you need a dramatic moment and you know you need it relatively soon and you know you need a resolution. There were times where we were absolutely frantic to get a section because we knew it was an aspect that was going to be covered. *Regardless of how frequently sections happen in the real world* we knew it was going to work for television.
>
> (Henderson, 2007: 116; emphasis added)

Producers recounted how people with mental illness were sometimes filmed 'performing for camera' and that these scenes were included occasionally due to financial constraints which meant that deadline pressures must be met and there was limited time for filming. At times the actual process of filming was believed to fuel 'patients' delusions:

> We were doing things that fed into their illness. Like one chap had delusions that he was paranoid and he completely felt that the hospital was out to get him and he was frightened to death and he thought he had hired this film crew to record every instance in order to keep the hospital on their toes. In some cases there were people who thought there were cameras in every room. There was one chap who thought that cameras were following him and the doctor said 'But they are!'
>
> (Henderson, 2007)

Independent producers were not exempt from pressure from senior management. Some producers recalled being forced to change the programme title or to rewrite the press release to ensure greater pre-transmission publicity. Underpinning these decisions was the desire to attract wider media interest (in previews). Some were advised by senior management to make material 'more shocking', with the implication that controversial television would attract greater audiences. The problem of what is considered to be 'televisual' becomes even more significant when producers discussed the challenge of portraying mental health. Indeed the same producers often struggled to find televisual moments in ongoing therapy sessions or to map the typical reality of mental distress where people might become well and then ill again. As one producer summarized, 'There were an awful lot of times when people were being fairly interestingly ill, then getting better, then more ill again so what we did in the editing was to generate narrative' (Henderson, 2007: 117). Producers recounted that portraying mental health was very difficult – typical images of someone walking in a park or making a cup of tea were considered to operate as cultural shorthand for 'normality' but clearly lacked the drama and pace of acute mental illness.

The documentary format has now proliferated in different directions and new media formats such as reality television programmes are considered to provide new possibilities for audience–producer relations (Hill, 2005). Popular programmes such as the *Big Brother* game show have generated youth audiences that are urgently required to generate advertising revenue. These programmes often generate controversy in terms of their sexual content, but in the UK Series 6 (Channel 4, 2006) the format was accused of promoting discrimination of people with mental illness. Within a few days of the new *Big Brother* season one participant left the programme after declaring to camera that he planned to self-harm.

The contestant in question, Shahbaz Choudhary, was pictured on the front page of the *Sun* newspaper under the headline 'I'll kill myself on telly' (23 May 2006). With unfortunate timing the celebrity gossip magazine, *Heat*, introduced the new contestants with a striking strap-line 'Unleash the mentalists' (23 May 2006). In the following days the ethical code of the programme was endlessly debated by website forum users and mental health charities and organizations. The Samaritans, the Mental Health Foundation and Sane expressed their condemnation of the programme for including such fragile characters. Complaint letters were sent to regulatory board Ofcom after the visibly shaken Choudhary appeared in front of a live audience on the spin-off programme *Big Brother's Little Brother* in which he told the presenter that he was unsure whether he would survive in the outside world.

Choudhary later revealed that he had lied about his mental health history to programme psychologists. Dr Andrew McCulloch, chief executive of the Mental Health Foundation, wrote an open and widely reported letter to Channel 4 saying:

> This kind of programming can make individuals who are distressed a laughing stock and this will only seek to feed the discrimination that already impacts heavily on people suffering from mental illness. It is disappointing that Channel 4 seems to have little regard for vulnerable contestants in the Big Brother house. I should be interested to know what screening and welfare measures are in place to protect contestants.
>
> (Brook, 2006)

However, Channel 4 denied that such contestants are exploited and maintained that there is a great deal of support that is 'hidden' from camera. John Corner (2002) speaks of a post-documentary age in which more serious documentary must be located within new forms of production and consumption. For Corner, programmes such as *Big Brother* offer what he terms 'a predefined stage precisely for personality to be competitively displayed (the intimate face to-camera testimony of the video room being one privileged moment) and for its "ordinary" participants to enter the celebrity system of popular culture with minimum transitional difficulty (we know them as performers already), if only for a brief period' (Corner, 2002: 264).

It cannot be assumed that these new media formats offer a better line to more positive representations. In some ways these increasingly voyeuristic television formats play on old stereotypes – viewers are encouraged to watch people behaving 'oddly'. Such controversies tend to increase viewer ratings and the economic importance of these programmes to the channel means that there may be priorities, which override ethical considerations.

Constructing the other: television drama

Television serial drama has become the focus for lobbying by a number of campaigners in the field of health and illness. Arguably, the ways in which mental health issues are presented in television fiction are equally if not more important in terms of audience beliefs (Henderson, 2007: ch. 5). These formats attract large and loyal audiences – millions of people watch a single episode of a soap opera or serial drama. Storylines are discussed in other media and are the topic of gossip and speculation, which means that they reach many more people than their actual audience (Henderson, 1999, 2007). Characters with mental illness depicted in entertainment media are frequently defined solely in terms of their illness (Sieff, 2003). Camera angles, as well as lighting and music, are believed to contribute to the signifying of 'dangerousness' of mentally ill characters in television drama (Wilson *et al.*, 1999). High-profile storylines have attracted criticism for depicting violent 'psychiatric patients'.

When, in 2000, the popular medical drama *ER* concluded its sixth series with the stabbing of two popular characters by a 'mentally ill patient' the programme was condemned by public health researchers. The report entitled 'The psychokiller strikes again' appeared in the *British Medical Journal* (Condren and Byrne, 2000). The authors condemned the programme unreservedly for misrepresenting the incidence of violent psychiatric patients. In earlier episodes of the same series a total of 28 other characters were identified who represented those with 'psychiatric problems', many of whom were violent (one man smashes his car because of 'demons', a child kills another child, a woman stalks a doctor). They concluded that 'the series, in making such a strong association between psychiatric illness and violence, is following established trends in television news, drama and the tabloid press. It is adding to the process of stigmatisation by the media' (Condren and Byrne, 2000).

The Glasgow Media Group study discussed earlier identified the power of television soap opera in which central characters were presented as 'mentally ill'. In one storyline in popular soap opera *Coronation Street*, a young Irish nanny is discovered to suffer from the condition 'erotomania' and in *Brookside*, a sexually violent husband and father attacks his family and is frequently referred to as a 'nutter' and 'psycho' both in the programme episodes and by wider media coverage of the storyline. These fictional stories were found to fuel existing public prejudice among audiences. However it is useful to briefly address how the characters were constructed. Interviews with scriptwriters and producers revealed that there was little commitment to the issue of mental illness (indeed neither production team believed that the story theme was one concerning mental illness).

The storyline in *Coronation Street* focused on themes of erotic obsession and drew on popular Hollywood cinema (specifically the popular film, *Fatal*

Attraction) to present audiences with a gripping drama in which 'Carmel' becomes obsessed by the father of the family who employ her. She pretends that she is pregnant and tells his wife that they are having an affair. Carmel was cast as 'fresh-faced' and 'angelic'-looking in order to maintain suspense for audiences. As the producer described: 'Carmel, the nanny from hell and stories like that [are very strong]. Where you get someone new like Carmel who introduces a catalyst into a happy family and suddenly it all sort of festers and turns bad. I mean there's a really good story' (quoted in Henderson, 1996: 23).

The production team at *Brookside* cast the character of 'Trevor' with similar concerns in mind and the story was constructed to 'keep audiences guessing' for as long as possible. The actor was known to British audiences from previous light comedy roles and this meant that his renewed violence and the shocking rape of his teenage daughter were all the more unexpected. As one writer describes, 'if you portray the baddie ... perpetrator from day one ... and you have no sympathy at all for him then people will just not engage in the story. You have to play against [the fact that] you know the audience will fall into the trap of 'he looks like a baddie therefore he must be one' (quoted in Henderson, 1996: 24).

The *Brookside* storyline showed Trevor as charming and friendly to neighbours while at the same time increasingly violent and volatile in the family home. Both of these storylines were incredibly popular with audiences (and indeed critics) yet played on existing misconceptions of people with mental illness (duplicitous, unpredictable, violent). Such storylines involving stalking, obsession and violence are familiar in television serial drama and, as noted earlier, these stories clearly reference Hollywood films (*Sleeping with the Enemy* and *Fatal Attraction* were both acknowledged as sources). Yet it is crucial to note that neither production team considered that they were covering a mental illness story. Perceptions of story theme are crucial in terms of how it will be constructed for audiences. Indeed, the BBC soap opera *EastEnders* attracted praise for its sensitive portrayal of Joe Wicks, a young character suffering from schizophrenia.

The mental health campaign organization MIND presented the programme with an award for the positive way in which this character had been developed. Significantly, the Story Editor had worked previously on BBC medical drama *Casualty* and was keen to develop a storyline, which could move away from the necessary medicalized focus of this genre to explore the implications of schizophrenia within a family. The television soap opera, with its continuing storyline and emphasis on family life, offered precisely this opportunity.

The characterization was based on advice from a professional adviser to the National Schizophrenia Fellowship. Dr Adrianne Revely, who later wrote of her experiences with the *EastEnders* team in the *British Medical Journal*. Revely highlights the dilemma for those who consult on storylines and the significant responsibilities such a role entails, not least to their professional colleagues:

> Advising EastEnders on their schizophrenia story should be highlighted in red ink on my curriculum vitae. Everyone has been impressed. I must really know my stuff if EastEnders used me as a source. Of course the downside is that every

jarring nuance of the story and every inaccuracy is laid at my door, and there have been plenty of inaccuracies. The basic story – Joe's initial diagnosis of psychotic depression and then the diagnosis of schizophrenia – remains true to life. I have begged for the storyline to include modern treatment with a limbic-selective antipsychotic, good response, return to normal life (see Harper, 2005), followed by scenes in which Joe experiences stigma. Stigma is a key issue that we want to be aired, and of course, the very fact that there is an EastEnders story at all is destigmatising. Schizophrenia is the last great stigma.

(Revely 1997: 1560)

There are a number of points to make here. First, that the sociocultural positioning of an issue has an impact on how it is likely to be portrayed in television drama (stories involving breast cancer were subject to meticulous care and attention over accuracy and visual representation). It would simply be wrong to assume that these characters were developed in such a way to deliberately fuel prejudice and misconceptions about those with mental illness. However, the characters' mental illness was used to structure a story on the theme of obsession and violence and intersected with existing public views about those who are mentally ill (as violent, duplicitous, 'split personality').

By contrast, the *EastEnders* story of Joe Wicks was from the outset perceived as 'doing mental illness' and was developed with care and sensitivity. Quite clearly, the consultant who represented the views of the *National Schizophrenia Fellowship* to the programme was impressed by their commitment to the issue and saw it as a positive challenge to public misconceptions. In other words television soap operas will not inevitably portray mental distress negatively. However, it seems clear that characters such as Carmel and Trevor, *regardless of the productions' intentions*, became part of a wider cultural repertoire of media images in which the mentally ill are demonized. The appropriation of conventions used in iconic Hollywood films can operate as important cultural signifiers for audiences and contribute to this process (see Henderson, 2007).

Media impact on audiences

Underpinning most of the studies discussed above is a serious concern with the impact of such media images on public understandings. However it is difficult to give a simple overview of audience research and mental illness. The techniques vary widely and it is hard to assess their generalizability. Rather than giving an overview of audience studies in the field, the audience reception strand of the Glasgow Media Group study of mental illness and the media will be discussed (Philo, 1996). This highlighted that audiences draw on images from factual and fictional media interchangeably.

The audience study involved groups of those without any obvious special knowledge or interest in mental illness ('general sample), as well as a series of interviews with users of services, their families and carers. A number of participants took part in focus groups where they were asked to write matching dialogue for photographs (taken from the *Coronation Street* story) or were given newspaper headlines (including the false report discussed earlier where a boy was reportedly 'set on fire') and asked to write a press report. The 'Carmel' story generated astonishing hostility. When people were asked how they would have reacted in the same situation as many as two-thirds of the sample gave responses that suggested aggression or violence. Typical responses included: 'Killed her, slapped her and called the police, punched her face in.' Far fewer responses related to more sympathetic care: 'she was unstable and needed some kind of help' (Philo, 1996: 92–3). In the second and third phase of the group sessions participants were asked about their beliefs and whether those people with illnesses such as schizophrenia were likely to be violent. Crucially, 40 per cent of people agreed that this was the case and gave the media as the source of their belief (Philo, 1996: 96). Participants drew on images from factual and fictional media interchangeably, as is suggested in the following quotation:

> A lot of things you read in the papers and they've been diagnosed as being schizophrenic. These murderers – say that Donald Nielsen, was he no schizo-phrenic? – the Yorkshire ripper ... in Brookside that man who is the child-abuser and the wife-beater – he looks like schizophrenic – he's like a split personality, like two different people. First he gets like self-pity and he brings flowers and works his way back into the house and you could feel sorry for him, then he's a child-abuser and a wife-beater.
>
> (Quoted in Philo, 1996: 96)

Other comments typically referenced popular culture sources in terms of how someone with schizophrenia might act: 'They could be alright one minute and then just snap – I'm kind of wary of them ... that *Fatal Attraction* she was as nice as ninepence and then ...' (quoted in Philo, 1996: 96). The issue of mental illness seemed to be a topic that was rarely discussed in family groups. Indeed, even where people had experience of people with mental illness through their professional work it did not necessarily mean that other members of the same family would hold the same belief. One woman worked as a matron in a hospital and had direct experience of people with mental illness. She did not asso-ciate them with violence; however, her three children did make this link. As her daughter wrote, 'Yes, I would say that people that have a mental illness would be violent. I have this idea as I have seen films about people with mental illnesses being murderers or violent. In newspapers it is always referred to a "psycho" killing someone' (Philo, 1996: 102).

It was also striking and in the context of audience reception research in other areas, highly unusual, that for some participants their own personal expe-rience was not enough to counteract powerful media images that linked mental illness with violence. For example, one woman gave the source of her belief as violent films such as *Nightmare on Elm Street* and *Psycho* but had direct experi-ence of visiting a relative in hospital who suffered mental illness. As she admits, 'I never saw any violence and he was in a big open ward.' Another woman asso-ciated mental illness with violence and split personalities but had worked on a fundraising event with 'patients' at a local mental hospital and found that none were violent. As she continues: "I remember being scared of them, because it was a mental hospital – it's not a very good attitude to have but it is the way things come across on TV, and films – you know, mental axe murderers and plays and things – the people I met weren't like that but that is what I associate them with' (quoted in Philo 1996: 104).

Interviews with service users reveal that media images are equally likely to affect them. One member of a user group in Manchester recalled how he felt before his diagnosis: 'I had the same misconceptions as everyone else, split personality, Jekyll and Hyde, flying off the handle at a second's notice, unpredictable, aggressive. [These came] partly from the family and possibly from what I'd seen on TV, radio, newspapers' (quoted in Philo, 1996: 109). A mother whose son was diagnosed with schizophrenia described being filled with guilt and anger at her misconceptions of the illness, 'I was working in a hostel with homeless and people would point at someone and say "he's schizo", and then I'd read something in the papers or see something on telly – that someone had killed someone or walked into a lion's den. I found out that schizophrenia wasn't split personality and that's only because of my son' (quoted in Philo, 1996: 109). Clearly a direct correlation between media representation and stigma is difficult to establish but the quotations above suggest that such media accounts can result in additional pain and distress for those coping in an already difficult situation.

Towards more balanced representations?

The aim of this chapter has been to highlight how mental illness is framed in different sections of the mass media. Many studies have identified that the links between mental illness and violence are promoted in the media at the expense of other more balanced or positive accounts. This is considered to be due to the lack of diversity in terms of sources, with the voice of the survivor remaining marginalized from mainstream media. New media formats provide opportunities for more challenging or critical representations yet sometimes become new forums for the airing of prejudice or exclusion. The perspectives of media professionals suggest that this negative profile is not deliberate but rather due to unspoken assumptions about what constitutes 'good television' or conforming to existing 'news values'.

Clearly the media has led the way in representing other groups who have been traditionally marginalized (gay and lesbian groups, ethnic minorities). Media campaigns have also engendered positive public awareness of other health and illness issues (HIV and AIDS, breast cancer) but we have yet to see this potential realized with the topic of mental health. It is crucial that those seeking to challenge media representation are aware of the factors that influence media practitioners. It is only with this 'media savviness' that practices can be successfully challenged. While there are no simple answers to how the media can be changed, adopting a more nuanced and finely targeted approach which recognizes and uses media diversity represents an obvious way forward.

▬▬▬▬▬▬▬▬▬▬▬ **EDITORS' QUESTIONS** ▬▬▬▬▬▬▬▬▬▬▬

Issues of difference

▧ Does the media depict mental illness differently for men and women?

▧ Consider if age is a barrier or incentive for filmmakers of people with a mental illness.

▧ Are cultural perspectives of mental health ever documented in the media?

Relevance to practice

▧ In what ways can scenes on television influence mental health professionals?

▧ How are mental health professionals depicted in the media?

▧ Identify the ways in which adverse media depiction of mental health professions can impact on individual practice.

Investigate

▧ Why do mental illness and crime receive high media attention?

▧ What are positive ways media can be used in highlighting the experiences of people with mental illness?

▧ How could mental health teams respond to negative images of mental illness?

Suggested Further Reading

Henderson, L. (2007) *Social Issues in Television Fiction*. Edinburgh: Edinburgh University Press.
Philo, G. (ed.) (1996) *Media and Mental Distress*. Harlow: Addison Wesley, Longman.

References

Aldridge, M. (1994) *Making Social Work News*. Routledge: London.
Brindle, D. (1999) Media coverage of social policy: a journalist's perspective. In B. Franklin (ed.) *Social Policy, The Media and Misrepresentation*. London: Routledge, pp. 39–50.
Brindle, D. (2006) New bill is leaner but many say meaner. *Guardian*, 22 November. Available online at www.guardian.co.uk.
Brook, S. (2006) Unhappy Shahbaz leaves Big Brother house. *Guardian*, 24 May.
Condren, R. and Byrne, P. (2000) The psychokiller strikes again (review). *British Medical Journal* **1282**: 320.
Corner, J. (1986) *Documentary and the Mass Media*. London: Routledge.
Corner, J. (2002) Performing the real: documentary diversions. *Television and New Media* **3**: 255–69.
Crepaz-Keay, D. (1996) A sense of perspective: the media and the Boyd Inquiry. In G. Philo (ed.) *Media and Mental Distress*. Harlow: Addison, Wesley, Longman, pp. 37–44.
Cross, S. (2004) Visualising madness: mental illness and public representation. *Television and New Media* **5**(3): 197–216.

DH (Department of Health) (1993) *The Ten Point Plan.* Press Release H93/908. London: Stationery Office.

DH (Department of Health) (1994) *Report of the Confidential Inquiry into Homicides and Suicides by Mentally Ill People (Boyd Report).* London: Stationery Office.

Ericson, R.V., Baraneck, P.M. and Chan, J.B.L. (1987) *Visualizing Deviance.* Milton Keynes: Open University Press.

Galtung, J. and Ruge, H.H. (1965) The structure of foreign news. *Journal of Peace Research* 2(1): 64–91.

Hallam, A. (2002) Media influence on mental health policy: long-term effects of the Clunis and Silcock cases. *International Review of Psychiatry* 14, 26–33.

Harper, S. (2005) Media, madness and misrepresentation: critical reflections on anti-stigma discourse. *European Journal of Communication* 20(4): pp. 460–85.

Henderson, L. (1996) Selling suffering: mental illness and media values. In G. Philo (ed.) *Media and Mental Distress.* Harlow: Addison Wesley, Longman, pp. 18–36.

Henderson, L. (1999) Producing serious soaps. In G. Philo (ed.) *Message Received.* Harlow: Addison, Wesley, Longman, pp. 62–81.

Henderson, L. (2007) *Social Issues in Television Fiction.* Edinburgh: Edinburgh University Press.

Hill, A. (2005) *Reality TV: Audiences and Factual Television.* London: Routledge.

Kilborn, R. (2003) *Staging The Real: Factual TV Programming in the Age of Big Brother.* Manchester: Manchester University Press.

Philo, G. (ed.) (1996) *Media and Mental Distress.* Harlow: Longman.

Philo, G., Henderson, L. and McLaughlin, G. (1993) *Mass Media Representations of Mental Health and Illness: Content Study.* Glasgow Media Group/Health Education Board for Scotland, Glasgow: Glasgow Media Group.

Philo, G. and Secker, J. (1999) Media and mental health. In B. Franklin (ed.) *Social Policy, The Media and Misrepresentation.* London: Routledge, pp. 135–45.

Plumb, A. (1993) The challenge of self-advocacy. *Feminism and Psychology* 3(2): 169–87.

Rassmussen, J. and Hoijer, B. (2005) *Media Images of Mental Illness and Psychiatric Care in Connection with Violent Crimes: A Study of* Dagens Nyheter, Aftonbladet *and* Rapport. Report for Swedish Association of Mental Health/Örebro University, Swedish Disability Federation/Umbrella Project. www.rsmh.se and www.paraplyprojektet.se

Revely, A. (1997) Soap tackles stigma of schizophrenia. *British Medical Journal,* **314**: 1560.

Schizophrenia home page (1997) Living with schizophrenia: EastEnders TV program covers schizophrenia [accessed 3/06].

Seale, C. (2002) *Media and Health.* London: SAGE.

Sieff, E.M. (2003) Media frames of mental illnesses: the potential impact of negative frames. *Journal of Mental Health* 12(3): 259–69.

Signorielli, N. (1993) *Mass Media Images and Impact on Health.* Westport, CT: Greenwood Press.

Wahl, O.F. (1995) *Media Madness: Public Images of Mental Illness.* New Brunswick, NJ: Rutgers University Press.

Wahl, O.F. (2003) News media portrayals of mental illness: implications for public policy. *American Behavioral Scientist* 46(1): 1594–1600.

Wahl, O.F., Wood, A. and Richards, R. (2002) Newspaper coverage of mental illness: is it changing? *Psychiatric Rehabilitation Skills* 6, 9–31.

Wilson, C., Nairn, R., Coverdale, J. and Panapa, A.I. (1999) Constructing mental illness as dangerous: a pilot study. *Australian and New Zealand Journal of Psychiatry* 33: 240–57.

Winston, B. (1995) *Claiming the Real: The Documentary Film Revisited.* London: BFI.

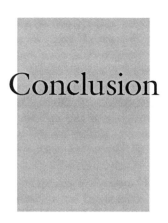

Conclusion

Tim Turner and Robert Tummey

As the ideas for this text began to take shape and develop, our vision was of a book that would stimulate debate around issues that are rarely questioned within the contemporary mental health system. While a diverse range of topics has been addressed within each of the preceding chapters, thematic threads are evident throughout the narrative.

The central message of the book is simple. As practitioners we are essentially part of a system that is flawed on almost every level. However uncomfortable we may find it, we operate within a pseudo-scientific framework that is founded on and perpetuates grossly unequal attributions of power (Szasz, 2007). Despite the rhetoric and benevolent veneer, each of us contributes to a system that creates and facilitates coercion, stigma, disempowerment, iatrogenic abuse and racism. Mental health provision continues to dehumanize those on the receiving end of treatment in a multitude of ways.

We have no doubt that the vast majority of mental health practitioners are well intentioned. The desire to help those in emotional distress is often the antecedent to a career within the mental health field. However, inevitably individuals slowly and subconsciously become immersed within the values, attitudes and assumptions of the system (Johnstone, 2000: 207). It is at this point that the issues addressed within these chapters become uncontested absolutes.

Our intention, then, was to offer practitioners some alternative angles on twenty-first-century mental health care; a fresh perspective. Although highly critical, the chapters are not awash with negativity. We encourage readers to think imaginatively, innovatively and reflexively about their roles. The content may seem to flow from the theoretical basis of anti-psychiatry. We prefer to think of it as post-psychiatry. Service users want a mental health system founded on equality, choice, self-advocacy, empowerment, respect and dignity (Read, 1996). If the balance of power is to be shifted, many of the issues highlighted within this textbook must be addressed. Mental health students may read the chapters with interest or scepticism at the various perspectives offered. All we suggest is they take a moment to reflect on the powerful influence they may exert within their practice and, when necessary, find the strength to challenge poor mental health care.

Can the system change? If individual practitioners critically reflect on their own practice and make the often small but meaningful changes, then perhaps the endemic culture of psychiatry can be gradually transformed. The first step along this road is the ability to cast a critical eye over the issues that permeate everyday practice.

Some time back, we discussed the prospect of creating a text that would draw these critical issues together in an accessible and thought-provoking way. Some practitioners may be uncomfortable with the opinions raised; psychiatry offers a position of power that is hard to relinquish. We hope you have taken something away from this book. At the very least we hope we have given you something to think about.

References

Johnstone, L. (2000) *Users and Abusers of Psychiatry* (2nd edn). London: Routledge.
Read, J. (1996) What we want from mental health services. In J. Read and J. Reynolds (eds) *Speaking Our Minds: An Anthology*. London: Open University Press.
Szasz, T. (2007) *Coercion as Cure*. London: Transaction.

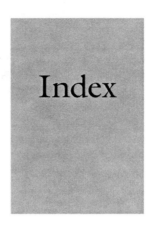

Index